EBURY PRESS

THE BOOK OF BODY POSITIVITY

Dr Rajeev Kurapati practices hospital medicine and holds the position of assistant professor of medicine at the University of Kentucky, USA. Triple-board certified, and specializing in obesity and lifestyle medicine, Rajeev is also the award-winning author of three books—*Unbound Intelligence* (2014), *Physician: How Science Transformed the Art of Medicine* (2018) and *Burnout in Healthcare* (2019). His writing has appeared in Slate, *Cincinnati Enquirer, Journal of Medical Economics*, Mind Body Green, Life Hack and Millennial Magazine.

Celebrating 35 Years of
Penguin Random House India

ADVANCE PRAISE FOR THE BOOK

'A trusted guide for those who struggle with losing weight'—Dr Deepti Behl, oncologist, Sutter Medical Center, Sacramento, California

'A must for those trying to understand the weight–food relationship at its core. Simply broken down and explained'—Dr Anna Fleytman-Pope, emergency medicine physician, Charlotte, North Carolina

'An honest and insightful description of the complex history of weight gain followed by a strategic guide to win the battle of weight loss'—Dr Liz Dulaney-Cripe, MD, orthopaedic surgeon, Ohio

The Book of Body Positivity

How We Got it All Wrong and What We Can Do About it

Dr Rajeev Kurapati

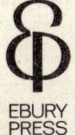

EBURY
PRESS

An imprint of Penguin Random House

EBURY PRESS

USA | Canada | UK | Ireland | Australia
New Zealand | India | South Africa | China | Singapore

Ebury Press is part of the Penguin Random House group of companies
whose addresses can be found at global.penguinrandomhouse.com

Published by Penguin Random House India Pvt. Ltd
4th Floor, Capital Tower 1, MG Road,
Gurugram 122 002, Haryana, India

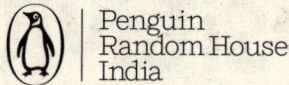

Penguin
Random House
India

First published in Ebury Press by Penguin Random House India 2023

ISBN 9780143461326

Typeset in Sabon by Manipal Technologies Limited, Manipal
Printed at Replika Press Pvt. Ltd, India

www.penguin.co.in

Contents

Disclaimer

The content of this book is for informational purposes only. It is not a substitute for professional medical advice. All patient names referenced in the book, as well as identifying events and places, have been changed to protect the privacy of individuals and their families.

Introduction

Obesity Is on the Rise—So Are Unrealistic Standards of Beauty

'Fat' is usually the first insult a girl throws at another girl when she wants to hurt her.

—J.K. Rowling

Have you ever experienced bullying for being overweight? Even if some remarks weren't blatantly cruel, have you ever felt that the 'jokes' were aimed at you?

If so, in all likelihood, you felt embarrassed or outraged, or maybe you endured the emotional ache silently. Perhaps you thought an overweight person deserves bullying—that *you* deserve bullying. After all, the weight has to come from somewhere. Surely weak willpower was involved. Right?

Even if you haven't experienced this yourself, you've likely seen or heard someone shame another person because they exist in a larger body. It's possible you too may have made someone feel shame for their body. As obesity rates skyrocket, so does the shaming of those affected by it. Rather than add to this message, it's time to turn the conversation in a different direction.

* * *

Fat shaming is the act of making fun of someone for being overweight or implying or stating that an overweight person is worthless, useless, lazy or even disgusting due to their size. It often manifests in the form of jokes made at an individual's expense or remarks about what and how someone eats, usually with implicit judgemental and insensitive undertones. The commonly held belief is that this may motivate people to eat less, exercise more and lose weight. However, bullying is typically malicious and cruel in nature. In most cases, people who fat shame have never struggled with a weight problem and don't fully understand the implications of their words (though this is no excuse for their behaviour).

Social media is a place people often turn to for support when they encounter bullying and stigma in the real world, but research shows that much of the discussion surrounding obesity on social media actually involves fat shaming as well, which often progresses into harassment and cyberbullying, particularly against women. In fact, there are entire online communities dedicated to making fun of overweight people, including sharing photographs of people obtained without their permission.

Among women, obesity-related stigma is now even more common than racial discrimination, according to the research carried out by Dr Rebecca Puhl and her colleagues at the Rudd Center for Food Policy and Health at the University of Connecticut.[1] Obesity stigma is a global phenomenon, with differences based on geography and culture. It is experienced by 19–42 per cent of adults, according to the World Obesity Report published on worldobesity.org. While the prevalence of obesity stigma is well documented in North America, France, Germany, the United Kingdom and Australia, evidence from other less studied countries, such as Argentina, Mexico, Paraguay, Puerto Rico, Tanzania and Qatar, is emerging. Obesity stigma is now recognized as a globalized health challenge.

* * *

Once upon a time, being heavy was a sign of wealth and prosperity while being thin was a sign of disease, ill health and poverty. Aesthetically, we have run the gamut of opinions surrounding weightiness—from the voluptuous, Rubenesque women of the seventeenth century to the heroine-chic supermodels of the twenty-first century.[2] The problem is, while aesthetic preference is one thing, modern media has glorified the tiny size-zero frame. At the same time, the obesity epidemic has surged and we're now in need of a conscientious assessment of who is responsible for this predicament.

Ethnographic studies comparing people's attitude towards large-sized individuals have shifted just in the past three decades. Research coming from Fiji conducted in the 1980s–90s described high value placed on voluptuous bodies but by the mid-2010s, large bodies were increasingly viewed as undesirable and uncontrolled. Another research study in the early 2000s from the Central American country, Belize, identified large, curvy-bodied women as attractive.[3] By 2015, the same population showed anti-fat sentiment where large bodies were seen as a social and economic liability.

In a 2013 survey conducted by Clear Voice Research entitled, 'Who Is to Blame for the Rise in Obesity?' and published in the journal *Appetite,* about 800 representatives of the US population were asked, 'Who is primarily to blame for the rise in obesity?' Respondents had to consider different entities—individuals, parents, farmers, food manufacturers, grocery stores, restaurants and government policies—and categorize them as 'primarily to blame', 'somewhat to blame' or 'not to blame' for the rise of obesity in America. The result of the study was shocking—it showed that 94 per cent of respondents believed individuals are at fault for the rise in obesity, i.e. obese people are *themselves* responsible for their weight.[4]

Is this an accurate and truthful conclusion? Objectively, it isn't. Are individuals entirely responsible for their weight? The answer is more complex than you may think, but the short answer is no, they aren't. If an individual isn't solely responsible, then who is?

In this book, I examine the stigma surrounding obesity, how that stigma came to be, and how it has been ingrained in our society and perpetuated through generations. I examine the role of the medical community in perpetuating this stigma, as well as the part doctors like myself and other healthcare professionals play in redefining what we deem to be healthy, and how we arrive at these conclusions. Finally, I outline current, evidence-based facts about obesity alongside suggestions for what we can do as a society to be more inclusive and less judgemental, while fostering an attitude towards health that is more concerned with what is going on *inside* the body than what it looks like on the *outside*.

Chapter 1 examines why we stigmatize obesity and what are its consequences. The stigma associated with obesity can be seen in every facet of our society, even among members of the medical community. Doctors, nurses and perhaps, most astonishingly, dieticians, have all been guilty of perpetuating the misconception that obesity is a personal failing. The impact of this stigma stops people who are affected by obesity from seeking help and receiving appropriate treatment, as well as deeply impacting their mental health, feelings of self-worth and self-confidence.

Chapter 2 explores how we define obesity (using body mass index or BMI) and what's wrong with it. Today's BMI methodology was adapted from the Quetelet Index—a tool developed by health insurance companies in the 1950s to justify an increase in their premiums based on weight. Unsurprisingly, BMI is fundamentally flawed as a means to diagnose obesity, as it doesn't measure actual fat content or fat quality (healthy fat vs sick fat). It also fails to take into account, race, ethnicity, gender or the lifestyle of the individual. For a compassionate and effective approach to tackling excess fat, we must re-evaluate the role of BMI, positioning it more as a preliminary screening tool rather than the definitive metric for obesity. Additionally, I urge the medical community to adopt 'adiposity' in place of 'obesity', centering the attention on fat tissue rather than an individual's overall size. In this chapter, I also explore why issues like metabolic dysfunction (such as insulin resistance and chronic inflammation) need to be addressed first, before obesity. If we fix the former, we fix the latter.

Chapter 3 examines why our body defends set-point weight and makes it hard to lose and maintain weight. Due to evolutionary design, our bodies have a 'set point', a weight at which we naturally tend to sit, give or take a few kilograms, that's maintained by multiple biological feedback control mechanisms. Many variables—from genetics to an individual's metabolism and gut microbiome—make it easy for them to gain weight and hard to lose it. This is why two people with the same diet and lifestyle may have entirely different body shapes and composition. Intermittent fasting and the 10 per cent solution, elaborated upon in great detail later, are two methods by which we can work against our body's set point.

Chapter 4 explores the psychosocial impact of weight-loss (bariatric) surgery. Just as there is a stigma surrounding obesity, there's one surrounding weight-loss surgery as well. While weight-loss surgery may be a necessary measure or last resort for someone in an acute health crisis, the psychological impact of bariatric surgery is significant and many people struggle after the procedure. Preparation for the surgery is intensive, and the post-op journey is long and demanding. While the surgery may be deemed 'successful' for some, others won't achieve the results they hope for. They may even gain back lost weight over time or suffer other complications.

Just as obesity is classified using the flawed BMI system, so is anorexia. Paradoxical as it may seem, an individual can meet all major diagnostical criteria for anorexia, but their weight can still fall within the range of being considered overweight or obese. This precludes patients from receiving treatment for an eating disorder they may desperately require. This is yet another way the stigma surrounding obesity has created a smokescreen around other underlying problems, preventing sufferers from accessing the appropriate treatment or help.

Chapter 5 delves into the intricate interplay between neurobiology and the environment, shedding light on the complexities underlying food addiction. The maladaptive compulsive overconsumption of food plays a large role in the rise of non-communicable diseases, of which obesity tops the charts. Obesity and its related diseases are considered to be the second leading cause of death, with the first being tobacco use. Smoking starts off as a choice and eventually becomes an addiction once the body gets habituated to the nicotine. We have contrived many ways to treat cigarette addiction, just as we have for other types of addiction, like alcohol and narcotic drug use. If obesity is due, at least partly, to an addiction to food, why don't we have ways to treat this type of addiction? What is food addiction really? And, perhaps most critically, who is responsible for it?

There is an idea deeply rooted in the scientific medical community that if something can't be fixed with a script pad or scalpel, it isn't treatable. Chapter 6 highlights two dominant hypotheses that drive our food consumption habits: calorie counting and low-fat diets, and how these two theories, although conceived (perhaps) with the right intentions by the founding researchers, are misused by the food industry to unscrupulously promote specific products—many of which actually contribute significantly to the global burden of obesity.

The manipulation of science and data by marketing companies to sell us unhealthy, calorie-dense, sugar-rich foods is a major contributing factor to the obesogenic world in which we now live. Unfortunately, this marketing often targets vulnerable populations, including those with fewer options or less access to healthier choices. Chapter 7 explores willpower and questions how much free will we really have in a world where our decisions are meticulously influenced by carefully crafted marketing.

People living in larger bodies have begun to push back against fat-shaming stigmas. Chapter 8 explores the impact of diet culture on our society and how it has shaped us to believe that thinner is always better. The body positivity movement and the 'Health at Every Size' movement are just two examples of ways people are advocating for greater levels of self-acceptance and self-love, irrespective of size or shape. These are sound concepts but they aren't perfect solutions.

Chapter 9 examines age-related weight gain. As we age, a variety of factors play into weight gain that makes it seem unavoidable. A little bit of weight gain as we age is normal, but if we aren't careful, that weight gain can become a catalyst for a host of other issues. There are many reasons for this phenomenon, some or all of which may contribute to an individual gaining substantial weight as they age and accelerating many other age-related illnesses. However, hope is not lost and there is much people can proactively do to stay within a healthy weight range for their specific needs, even at an advanced age.

The final chapter examines the role of governmental policies in either curbing the rising rate of obesity or contributing to it. Ultimately, obesity is never a reflection of an individual's motivation, drive or willpower. These facts are presented in this book to spark further conversation around some of the biggest and most damaging misconceptions surrounding obesity, with the hope of mitigating the stigmatization and discrimination that targets individuals because of their size or weight.

* * *

1

Why Do We Stigmatize Obesity and What Are the Consequences?

We expect medical professionals to be the experts on issues related to health. Regrettably, when it comes to obesity, most of them are mistakenly conditioned to equate larger body sizes with adiposopathy. Sick fat disease or adiposopathy is a pathological process responsible for many metabolic diseases. The outward appearance, i.e. obesity (defined by BMI) is merely a *symptom* of such a dysfunctional cellular process. A conscientious medical expert recognizes the distinction between the pathological process and its symptoms while understanding their interrelation, and recommends treatments accordingly. But unfortunately, we are habituated to judging a person's health based on their size. It is no surprise that the metrics and tactics we use to define and combat adiposity aren't working.

People from different ethnicities and cultures come in different sizes and shapes.[1] Some are fleshier while others are leaner. Some are top-heavy, others are rotund. We cannot define a universal 'normal size' body for everyone globally, and it is absurd and incorrect to try to make them fit into that size. Even if everyone ate identical meals and followed the same exercise regime every day, our bodies would look and function differently. Bigger body size doesn't automatically translate to sickness.

* * *

'Why does everyone want to talk about my weight?' asked my patient, Cathy. As I took a breath and paused, she snarled at me before I could answer. 'Honey, I'm not here to discuss that. I'm here because I have an infection in my leg. Just take care of it and let me go.' She was enraged and adamant.

Cathy was an African American woman in her late fifties. She was admitted to the hospital three days earlier for cellulitis, a bad infection of the skin and subcutaneous tissue in her right leg. She was prescribed IV antibiotics for about two weeks. The infection started as a small pimple after she bumped her little toe against a door. It spread slowly and insidiously until her entire leg was red, swollen and painful. She decided to come to the emergency room when the pain became unbearable.

Her life had turned upside down when her spouse died in an accident. She packed up everything, and, together with her children, she relocated to Kentucky, where her parents lived. Due to her circumstances, she raised her children as a single mother and a grieving widow.

After she relocated, Cathy purposefully avoided establishing care with a new primary physician. Every time she made an appointment, the first thing the doctor would advise her was to lose weight, regardless of the purpose of her visit, whether it was for a urinary tract infection or an annual exam. Rather than having her medical concerns addressed, the doctors were convinced that her weight was the sole reason for her health problems. She claimed that they disregarded and invalidated her, putting her in an indefinite state of hurt because of her size. Cathy told me that the staff at the doctor's office would 'physically recoil' upon seeing her.

'Sometimes, the doctor refuses to examine me because he doesn't want to touch me,' she said in a husky, tear-clotted voice.

She added that on several occasions, doctors went as far as issuing an ultimatum: lose weight or she won't get another visit at that office. 'But, how can I?' she inquired. 'I've always been a big girl, and doctors often tell me to eat less and exercise more, as if I haven't already done that. Nobody ever informs me what to do next or expect, when I exercise but don't lose weight.' Her tone grew louder, her remarks expressing a genuine sense of rage and hurt stemming from years of torture. 'They assume I'm a slacker or unconcerned about myself. So, I simply stopped going to the doctors.'

We may have just met a few minutes ago, but I could immediately feel the weight of the injustice she had experienced. At that moment, I recalled a story I had recently read in the newspaper of a young Californian woman who—despite repeatedly seeking care—was told time and again by doctors that losing weight was the solution to her worsening symptoms. It turned out that her symptoms were due to an undiagnosed advanced bone marrow cancer. Her story doesn't exist in isolation either. Every day, many people suffer from undiagnosed diseases and therefore go untreated because the first thing their doctor sees is a high BMI.

'I'm truly sorry to hear you've faced such experiences,' I remarked. Moving forward, I asked, 'How have you been adhering to your medications for diabetes and high blood pressure?'

'I stopped taking them,' she responded. 'I bought some vitamins and started eating better, hoping that I wouldn't have to visit the doctor again for a while. Unfortunately, here we go again.' She looked down at the tile floor resignedly, and her bold and strong voice abated. The room went quiet.

* * *

Weight Stigma in Healthcare Setting

The stigma surrounding plus-sized patients is pervasive and is regrettably exacerbated by medical professionals. In a study entitled 'Primary Care Physicians' Attitudes about Obesity and Its Treatment', researchers analysed 620 physicians' responses to a questionnaire. They concluded that 'physicians view obesity largely as a behavioural problem and share the broader society's negative stereotypes about their attributes of obese persons'.[2]

Simply put, despite their medical training, healthcare professionals judge and stigmatize obese individuals as much as the general public does.

Numerous studies analysed overweight and obese individuals in their respective healthcare settings to understand more about existing biases towards weight. It was found that healthcare settings are, in fact, a significant source of discrimination. In a 2006 survey, heavy individuals were asked to rank the possible sources of obesity bias in order of frequency. It turned out that physicians were rated the second most common, with family members topping the list. Younger obese women reported more stigma compared to their older counterparts. The same study reported that half of the women received inappropriate comments from their physicians regarding their weight.[3]

Research also shows that discrimination touches all disciplines in the field. Weight stigmatization has been documented among dieticians and even mental health specialists. This stigma significantly deters obese patients from seeking and receiving the medical care they need and deserve.

In another study, obese participants reported that they avoid booking a future appointment with the clinic because they fear that their physician will reproach them if they have gained weight recently.[4]

Sadly, this bias developed even before the medical professionals stepped into their official roles. Both self-reported and experimental research showed that obese and overweight patients were labelled, stereotyped and discriminated against by medical students, including the views that obese patients are lazy, unmotivated, dishonest, ignorant and non-compliant with suggested treatment.

In a 2009 study published in the *Journal of Clinical Nursing*, groups of nursing students and registered nurses perceived obesity negatively. The majority of nursing staff found obese individuals 'shapeless, slow and unattractive'. Half of the questionnaire's participants felt that obese adults should be put on a diet while in the hospital. More alarmingly, registered nurses displayed more of such negative biases than students.[5] This indicates that negative stereotypes were internalized from a young age when the students were still undergoing medical training and continued throughout their professional careers.

In addition, research also revealed that healthcare providers assign less time to obese or overweight patients, build less of a rapport with them and offer fewer educational resources compared to patients of average weight. Studies have shown that even doctors, nurses and nutritionists often overestimate the actual food intake of heavy people.

Due to the gross disrespect these patients feel, along with the feelings of inadequacy and a sense that their health concerns are deliberately neglected, many patients harbour resentment and distrust towards healthcare professionals. Needless to say, this makes patients hesitant or even unwilling to discuss their weight with any medical professional. They might just avoid healthcare settings altogether like Cathy.

Unfortunately, many healthcare professionals are oblivious to their own deep-rooted biases towards heavier patients. Until we address this implicit bias directly within the medical community, educate healthcare professionals and encourage them to question their preconceptions towards their obese patients, the cycle of stigma from healthcare professionals and their mistreatment of patients will continue.

Stigma in Society

In 2021, a multinational study exploring weight bias in six countries polled adults from Australia, Canada, France, Germany, the UK and the US. The results highlighted the adverse effects of weight prejudice on healthcare habits and experiences, emphasizing the urgency for a united international response to this issue.[6]

In his 1968 article 'The Stigma of Obesity', American sociologist Werner Cahnman, through a series of gradated interviews at an obesity clinic in a low-income New York neighbourhood, observed that the discrimination towards young overweight patients is crippling to their sense of self and creates shame from which they 'cannot free themselves'.[7]

Rather than improving over time, the landscape is grimmer today. In support of Cahnman's findings, psychologist Janet Tomiyama observed in a 2018 study that obesity stigma is now 'more socially acceptable, severe and sometimes more prevalent than racism, sexism, and other forms of bias'.[8] These stigmas are not separate; they are interwoven threads in the web of discrimination. While one can exist on its own, the presence of more than one of these stigmas only serves to compound the oppression and prejudice the person in question faces. This finding illustrates that today, we judge people based on weight and social status. It also illustrates the emphasis on appearance in our modern society and its impact on a person's overall well-being when they don't fit within the supposed 'average'.

The stigma compounds in other ways as well. Studies show that people subjected to persistent negative stereotypes have a higher risk of developing heart disease and diabetes. When such weight-based stigma gets under their skin, they internalize the pain, profoundly affecting themselves mentally and psychologically. The prejudice these individuals experience increases their likelihood of developing obesity-related illnesses in the future.

Stigma at Home, School and at the Workplace—No Place Is Safe from Discrimination

In a Brazilian survey of 3621 people with obesity, 72 per cent of respondents reported that family environment is the most hostile environment when it comes to shaming linked to their weight.[9]

Stigma at home can be more traumatic than in any other setting. Home is meant to be a haven, a safe space where one can retreat from the harshness and challenges of the external world. The pain of being labelled and degraded by your closest family members can erode someone's self-esteem and their view of themselves. Though nicknames like 'pudgekins' or 'thunder thighs' from your mother or siblings may be portrayed as terms of endearment, they serve as constant, subconscious reminders that you are being judged, no matter how acceptable it may be for you.

The damage is beyond just a blow to an individual's self-esteem. A 2018 study titled, 'Adolescents' Perspectives on Everyday Life with Obesity', revealed that obese adolescents felt uncomfortable and stigmatized when attention was drawn to their weight. With good intentions, the families adopted behavioural avoidance techniques to counteract this. Unfortunately, this inevitably led to a pervasively hostile home environment, particularly around mealtimes, with family members treading on eggshells, afraid to offend the adolescent. Although well intentioned, avoiding the topic generated an uneasiness that transformed the home from being a place of safety, honesty and support to one of unease, tension and discomfort.[10] It has been proven that meaningful social support is a critical success factor in lasting weight loss. What is a better opportunity to provide meaningful social support than within the home?

Aubrey Gordon, author of *What We Don't Talk About When We Talk About Fat*, is a writer, blogger and podcaster who published under the alias, 'Your Fat Friend'. She has dedicated her life to battling the stigma of obesity. With a loyal and engaged group of followers across her social media platforms, she frequently addresses the experiences of moving through the world as a fat woman.

On her Twitter account, she asked her followers to share their experiences at home or with family members that drew attention to their weight and made them feel self-conscious or uncomfortable. One respondent wrote,

'In India, it's extremely common to call fat people "moti" (mo-tee), especially your family members. It translates directly to fat (in Hindi) and is a synonym for [an] elephant. I have been subjected to this for my entire life until today, especially by my immediate family, despite warning them not to do it. Their defense is that they say it out of love.'

This respondent's experience isn't unique—similar dialogues occur in hundreds of thousands of households worldwide. These comments hurt, even if (or precisely because) they come from loved ones. It's crucial to recognize that the remarks made about someone during their formative years can profoundly shape their self-perception and understanding of their role in the world for a lifetime.

For a child or adolescent who lives in a morally damaging home environment, school often becomes their refuge. Or does it? Sadly, for overweight children, school is not a relief from stigma as well. It might begin with taunts on the school bus and continue into the classroom or extracurricular activities. Another of Gordon's Twitter respondents, a woman now in her thirties, said, 'I was called a butterball. Kids would throw cookies at me on the school bus. It still hurts.' Even two decades later, she claimed that the pain, humiliation and rejection from the bullying she endured as a child still hurts her.

Undoubtedly, these behaviours are incredibly harmful. As they grow older, the perpetrators of these acts continue to stigmatize heavier people, where they will most likely be just as biased. Meanwhile, the affected children will grow into adulthood with the same trauma.

Bonita, a Mexican schoolteacher, shared how she was addressed unapologetically as 'Gordo' in the staff room, which means fat in Spanish. Almost the entire faculty called her by that nickname within a couple of weeks into her job. While we know that women tend to receive far more criticism for their appearance than their male counterparts, men are neither immune to slurs about their physical appearance nor unhurt due to such uninvited comments.

Regrettably, discrimination in the workplace goes beyond name-calling. A 2013 study conducted in Canada discovered that 45 per cent of employers were less inclined to recruit an overweight candidate due to the stigma associated with this demographic.[11] Virgie Tovar, an author and expert on fat activism, says that fatphobia has severely stunted her career growth. She once went through several rounds of interviews with very positive feedback. However, she was unexpectedly rejected for the job when she reached the final round of interviews with the manager at the San Francisco office. 'I go upstairs and I'm greeted at the elevator by a male, and he looked at me up and down and is visibly dissatisfied,' she says, believing she was a front runner for the post.[12]

Overweight and obese people were also offered a lower salary than peers who belonged to the 'acceptable' weight range. A research article from 2010 in the *Journal of Applied Psychology* discovered that women significantly heavier than the 'average weight' earned $19,000 less annually in the US, whereas notably slender women had an increased annual income of $22,000 compared to their average-weight counterparts. On average, an increase in weight by 25 pounds (11 kg) resulted in a yearly reduction of $14,000 in salary.[13] People affected by obesity are literally paying for their condition, which is very often beyond their control in the first place.

Though life may be easier in many instances for someone who falls within a more 'typical' weight range, no one is immune to the toxicity surrounding our culture's unrealistic expectations about weight and appearance. Most of our standards of beauty are derived from what we see every day in the media, on Instagram, the celebrities we see in movies and on television, or the musicians, artists and other influential figures who dominate the public eye. These people are under enormous pressure to look their absolute best in each moment, even when caught unaware by the paparazzi. They employ a team of nutritionists, chefs, personal trainers, private hairdressers and make-up artists, often undergoing expensive surgeries to achieve and maintain their appearance. It is ludicrous to expect ordinary people to achieve the same level of perfection.

Appearance-Based Stigma and Physical Deviance

In 1980, Dr William DeJong conducted an experiment where participants were given a photograph and asked to form a positive or negative first impression about the individuals depicted. The results showed that individuals who presented as obese needed to have a justification for their weight—some physiological condition out of their immediate control, such as a hormonal disorder—before they were viewed positively.[14] This is a concerning trend that shows no signs of wavering.

Our society has little to no concept of a healthy, sustainable lifestyle. On a daily basis, we are presented with images of extremes that most people cannot (and should not) emulate. Dieting, extreme workouts, a year-round tan, a blindingly white smile, lip fillers, boob jobs, butt lifts, expensive hair extensions, fake nails, fake eyelashes, hair plugs, bulging biceps and washboard abs—our culture has become unhealthily obsessed with outward appearance. Every degree a person deviates from this 'ideal appearance' is a moral fault.

Researchers Puhl and Brownell observed in their 2006 article titled, 'Confronting and Coping with Weight Stigma: An Investigation of Overweight and Obese Adults', that people consider obesity a form of physical deviance resulting from deviant behaviour akin to lying, child abuse or infidelity.[15, 16] This extremely demonizing belief persists despite the prevalence of scientific evidence, which supports a variety of factors entirely outside of an overweight individual's control. Despite this, the belief in personal control over someone's weight prevailed.

The Double-Edged Sword of Obesity

People affected by sick fat disease suffer at two levels—the first is their outward appearance due to the underlying disease as they wear their malady on their sleeve. The second is the disease itself.

Many diseases attributed to obesity such as hypertension, diabetes and even many cancers, slowly develop over the years, revealing themselves in unexpected bursts. Barriers to consistent, validating healthcare access reinforce the inescapability of these hidden conditions. As a result, many people slip through the cracks till it's too late.

Our assumptions about who is at fault, when laid bare, are shamefully present in every recess of society. Obesity is attributed to an individual's lack of knowledge, effort or willpower.

Before a disease ever had a scientific meaning, it had a social connotation. The construct that ill health is the result of personal shortcomings, and that we, as individuals, are solely accountable for our misery is deeply rooted in the human psyche. It is almost inextricable from the story of humanity. This seemingly old-fashioned attitude is still prevalent today, especially when we ostracize HIV patients, those with mental health conditions, those affected by addiction and, of course, people who are obese.

To end the social exclusion faced by people with adiposity, we need to change our attitudes, fill the knowledge gaps and reframe our thinking. Once we do that, we can begin to cultivate an environment where people affected by obesity want to and will be entitled to care without the fear of prejudice or dismissal. By simply identifying adiposity as a medical illness similar to any other, we have the power to alter the course of millions of people's lives worldwide. Every person deserves to live a life free from stigma and social condemnation, and we have the capacity to enhance people's quality of life, support their physical and mental health, and empower them to explore new avenues.

At a Glance

❖ Healthcare professionals promote our broader society's negative stereotypes about the personal attributes of obese persons.

❖ The social stigma associated with obesity affects people physically, mentally and psychologically.

❖ Research shows that society likens obesity to physical deviance, comparable to other deviant behaviour such as to lying, child abuse or infidelity.

❖ Overweight and obese people earn less money than peers who fall in an 'acceptable' weight range.

❖ To end the stigma regarding obesity, we need to change our attitudes, fill the knowledge gaps and reframe our thinking.

* * *

2

Your (Average) Doctor Knows Very Little about Adiposity

The term obesity was derived from the Latin word obesus, meaning 'that has eaten itself fat'.

Okinawans, once hailed as one of the world's healthiest communities, are now experiencing higher BMI rates, even higher than their Japanese mainland counterparts. Pacific islanders of Australia and New Zealand, who were known for their active lifestyles centred around farming, fishing and hunting, are now communities with the highest obesity rates worldwide. Despite the most advanced medical care, worldwide obesity has nearly tripled since 1975.[1] So how did obesity become such a serious problem in medicine? Are our methods at fault? Or did we incorrectly understand the obesity problem itself in the first place?

For centuries, no one knew how to measure it but we intuitively knew that fat has something to do with our health. Our ancestors knew that loss of plumpness in a child is associated with undernutrition and excessive fat is a sign of poor health. The irony is that we didn't know then, and don't know now, how much fat is healthy for the proper functioning of our body. The watershed moment in the history of nutritional medicine happened in 1972 when Ancel Keys proposed a new measurement to estimate body fat in populations. Epidemiologists fell in love with this metric and got married to this flawed tool, so much so that it became the gold standard in obesity medicine.

A doctor's fee for the disease of abnormal fat is tied to the diagnostic codes based on this metric. All epidemiological studies in nutrition science are based on BMI as a measure of obesity. Pharmaceuticals, weight-loss surgeries, the slimness industry and everything related to fatness are linked to this metric. Chasing BMI has become a preoccupation for many medical professionals, nutritionists, exercise specialists, epidemiologists and the weight-loss industry where thousands of research papers, dozens of pills, scores of procedures and millions of books and self-help programmes are thriving. Despite this, the rate of obesity continues to soar to astronomical proportions.

* * *

Defining Adiposity—Chasing the Wrong Target

Apex establishments like the World Health Organization (WHO) and Obesity Medicine Association (OMA) define obesity as an increase in body fat that promotes adipose tissue dysfunction and abnormal fat mass resulting in adverse metabolic, biomechanical and psychosocial health consequences.[2]

If you notice carefully, these definitions of obesity do not directly mention one's body size, shape or weight. However, in both medical practice and society, the most accepted measure of obesity is based on body size, appearance and weight. We define obesity by BMI, which is the ratio of a person's mass (kilograms) to his/her height squared (metres squared). Based on the BMI, an individual can be classified into five categories: underweight, normal, overweight, obese and extremely (or morbidly) obese.

The irony is that while obesity is defined as an abnormal or excessive fat accumulation, BMI, the unspoken gold standard used to diagnose adiposity, does not assess the body's fat percentage, function or distribution. Moreover, BMI doesn't account for age, sex, ethnicity or a person's lifestyle.

As a one-size-fits-all metric, BMI perpetuates a commonly accepted definition of adiposity that fails to assess the condition accurately. How then did we come to accept BMI as a universal measure of adiposity in the first place? The answer can be found by asking a more pertinent question: where did this faulty metric originate from and how did it gain widespread acceptance?

We don't have the faintest idea how to describe obesity in a way that encompasses all facts of the disease, let alone the suffering it causes.

The Replacement of Infectious Diseases with Diseases of Lifestyle

Back in the days when infectious diseases were responsible for most human deaths, thinness aroused concern, whereas plumpness and roundness were a sign of good health. While medical professionals struggled to determine the appropriate weight to be used as a health indicator, the insurance industry was quick with their answer—height and weight tables, i.e. correlating an 'ideal' weight for a particular height.

The 1950s was a watershed period in the history of medicine.[3] Thanks to improved standards of hygiene and sanitation, antibiotics and the introduction of vaccinations, infectious diseases accounting for most deaths in the US, such as tuberculosis, polio, malaria and intestinal infections, were successfully brought under control. While the rates of infectious diseases in the general population had declined, more patients suffered from non-infectious diseases, predominantly heart diseases and cancers. Even before these non-communicable conditions dominated the medical landscape, body weight was important for medical assessment. Insurance companies viewed extremes of weight as undesirable, often resulting in policy denial or significantly higher premium payments.

The premiums paid by the policyholders play a great role in the profitability of life insurance businesses.[4] A healthy policyholder is more likely to live longer (hence they pay smaller premiums over a longer duration). In contrast, a sick policyholder is required to pay a greater premium to cover the potential insurance claim in case of sickness or untimely death. Insurance companies needed a standardized and foolproof measurement to identify high-risk individuals quickly.

In the early days of the life insurance business, to determine whether an applicant would be granted a policy, companies hired doctors who would simply eyeball the applicant to conclude if they were of healthy weight or not.[5] Since no reliable standards (or metrics) were available back then to determine what was a healthy weight, the doctor's judgement was often proven inaccurate. As a result, the decision of such physicians became a costly mistake for many insurance companies.

The 'Average' Man

In the early 1830s, Belgian statistician Lambert Adolphe Quetelet suggested the idea of a height and weight table, even though its practical application came much later.[6] Quetelet sought to apply his knowledge of probability calculus to study trends in human populations. He was the first to conduct a cross-sectional growth study of Belgian newborns and children based on their height and weight, which later expanded to include adults. He discovered that weight increases as a cube of the baby's height during the first year of life and then shifts to a square of the height. As a result, he theorized that weight grows as a function of the square of height in adults, a concept known as the Quetelet Index. His observations were published in the book *A Treatise of Man and the Development of His Aptitudes*, released in 1835.

For nearly 140 years, this index lacked clinical application. However, a simultaneous concept introduced by Quetelet revolutionized population research in medicine.[7] Quetelet, who spent his life researching hidden patterns in populations, devised a method for combining separate measurements into a single aggregate metric to study the physical characteristics of individuals in a population. This concept of measuring averages gained popularity among his contemporaries.

Quetelet believed that when individual variations were averaged out, one could arrive at a profile of the 'average man' that would be representative of the population. This figure would be characterized by the mean values of all the measured attributes of people in a given population.

A British surgeon named John Hutchinson used this concept of averages to study the heights and weights of 2650 English men in order to devise a precise and easy method of detecting lung disease in populations. In his 1846 paper, eleven years after the conception of Quetelet's Index, Hutchinson created a table showing the average weight of individuals for each inch of height from 5'1" to 6' at the age of thirty. This height–weight chart became the standard for the British population and life insurance firms quickly took advantage of this tool to assess policy applicants' health status.

The 'Ideal' Weight

The Mutual Life Insurance Company of New York took the British reference table and applied it to the

North American population in 1867, twenty years after life insurance firms adopted Hutchinson's height–weight charts.[8] For the next forty-five years, a series of adjustments were made to the height–weight tables to standardize them. By 1912, a new concept called 'ideal' weight for a particular height was introduced into the language of population statistics.[9] The ideal body weight for a given height was defined as the optimal weight associated with the maximum life expectancy; 20–25 per cent above the ideal weight for a given height was deemed 'too fat'. Since then, all major life insurance companies across America have adopted this revised height–weight chart.

By this time, insurance companies using size as a health indicator had inadvertently influenced how the textile and fashion industries advertised their products. While policyholders could be classified by gender, height and weight, the numbers couldn't be grouped into a normal distribution curve until insurance researchers devised a brilliant solution: divide the population into body frames. This concept created a universally accepted standard for body proportions: extra small (XS), small (S), medium (M) and large (L). More frames were added as the population became larger: extra-large (XL), double extra-large (XXL), triple extra-large (XXXL), etc.

With the development of organized medicine and the incorporation of scientific research into the field, the medical community began to take an active role in modifying and transforming the ideas set forth by the insurance industry. These height–weight charts gained such popularity that doctors, dieticians, media and the general public began to accept them unconditionally.

The charts gained an unquestionable reputation for being dependable in evaluating what weight was normal or abnormal. The average weights assumed many names— 'normal' weight, then 'standard' weight, followed by 'ideal' weight—all in the insurance industry's attempt to find the weight that was optimal for their bottom line. These terms gradually became part of our collective consciousness and paint an impression that everyone falling outside of that 'ideal' weight is less healthy by default, probably the best example of one-size-fits-all.

From the Quetelet Index to the Body Mass Index

Ancel Keys (1904–2004), an American physiologist working at the University of Minnesota, was disgusted by the problem of corpulence and called it 'ethically repugnant, uncomfortable, and impeding motion . . . hard on clothes and furniture'.[10] He was one of the most influential figures in human nutrition studies during the 1970s. When his research subjects questioned how they could tell whether they were too fat, he was caught lecturing: 'If you want to know whether you are obese, just undress and look in the mirror. Don't worry about our complicated laboratory tests; you'll figure it out!' He wasn't naturally hostile to persons of large stature; he was deeply frustrated by the growing rate of obesity.

Instead of relying on the height–weight charts popularized by insurance companies, Keys conjured up a clever idea. He resurrected the long-forgotten Quetelet Index in his 1972 article by giving it a new name that stuck, the BMI.[11] At the time, Keys understood the limitations of using the formula to measure body fat. He said, 'If not fully satisfactory, at least the index is as good as any other relative weight index as an indicator of relative obesity.' Despite Keys' clear caution that BMI should only be applied to population-based studies and not for individual diagnoses, it nevertheless became a standard tool for categorizing individuals as underweight, overweight or obese. This metric gained universal acceptance, from epidemiologists' minds to doctors' offices.

In 1973, the Fogarty International Centre Conference on Obesity recommended the creation of a 'desirable range' of weight for a particular height based on size, i.e. BMI.[12] This idea had already been floated by the Metropolitan Life Insurance Company earlier in 1959 concerning the association between body weight and cardiovascular disease. When the US Department of Agriculture (USDA) and the US Department of Health, Education, and Welfare published their first edition of nutritional 'Dietary Guidelines for Americans' in 1980, they adopted the weight tables based on the Fogarty International Centre Conference on Obesity.[13] Newer terms were introduced. Overweight is above the 85th percentile of average BMI and obesity is above the 95th percentile. These definitions became widely accepted across all platforms as a standard index. Little attention was placed on the true problem that characterizes obesity: abnormal body fat percentage, fat composition and fat distribution.

In the third publication of the USDA 'Dietary Guidelines for Americans' released in 1990, a guideline issued every five years, 'desirable' weight was translated into numbers based on the BMI. In 1995, the WHO Expert Committee published a report called 'The Use and Interpretation of Anthropometry', which classified different levels of BMI into cut-off points.[14] Three years later, an expert panel convened by the National Institute of Health (NIH) in 1998 utilized the BMI to define the terms 'overweight' and 'obesity'.[15] Since then, public health professionals and epidemiologists have unconditionally settled on using BMI as the uncontested surrogate to assess adiposity. They accepted this imprecise but easier metric to conduct their research and convinced everyone in the medical community to do the same.

By using BMI as a tool to measure the degree of adiposity in large populations, disease-tracking scientists could predict several correlations between higher BMI and adverse health conditions. For instance:

1. A BMI above forty is linked to a reduction of ten years in life expectancy, comparable to smoking effects.[16]
2. A BMI greater than thirty doubles the risk of heart failure.
3. 80 per cent of all type 2 diabetes cases have a BMI in the obesity range.
4. A five-unit increase in BMI increases the risk of stroke by 20 per cent.
5. A BMI greater than thirty is associated with 230 comorbidities, including cancer.

Epidemiologists and nutrition researchers established an association between a high BMI and poor health outcomes. Professional medical organizations then based many dietary recommendations and preventive measures with BMI as the standard metric for adiposity. The entire medical community was convinced that adiposity and adiposopathy could be measured by BMI and all efforts had to be spent on driving this metric into an arbitrary range. Despite all their efforts, the rates of obesity never slowed down and no one knew where we went wrong.

Everyone across professional and non-professional sections of society was distracted by a metric that showed a *correlation* (between high BMIs and poor health outcomes) and failed to ask the question: What is it about higher BMI that *causes* these health problems?

For over half a century, population researchers' love affair with BMI steered the entire medical profession and the public into a blind alley by convincing us that adiposity is synonymous with a larger size. All along, we took our eyes off the real problem: adiposity and adiposopathy have more to do with dysfunctional fat tissue and less with the size of the person.

The Failings of BMI

The most serious flaw in using body size as a surrogate for adiposity measurement is its limitation in assessing body fat. Multiple studies advocate that body size alone cannot define adiposity, which is characterized not by excess weight but by excess fat mass and fat in the wrong places. BMI and other anthropometric measurements fail to distinguish between fat, muscle tissue, skeletal tissue and fluid weight. Muscle tissue weighs significantly more than fat tissue, meaning that many athletes are considered overweight or obese despite being in peak physical health.

Although studies have shown that a population's health risk increases as BMI increases, it cannot be used to measure an individual's adiposity. While individuals classified as obese often have excess body fat, and those in the obesity range might generally be less healthy, it's possible for someone to be obese yet metabolically healthy. Conversely, people with a BMI in the 'healthy' weight range can still have excess body fat affecting their metabolism. Thus, BMI classifications do not provide precise delineations between healthy and unhealthy weights.

BMI, while a quick and convenient metric for population research, should not be viewed as the sole indicator of individual adiposity, as even Ancel Keys has noted. Despite its limitations, many epidemiologists and policymakers still endorse it. The American Association of Clinical Endocrinologists, for instance, has issued somewhat conflicting guidelines regarding BMI's use in determining obesity. While they rightly suggest that BMI should initiate further adiposity evaluations, their guidelines also recommend using BMI to confirm and classify individuals as overweight or obese after additional assessments, factoring in age, gender, ethnicity, fluid status and muscle mass.[17]

The irony of such statements, endorsing BMI as a screening tool and at the same time, a confirmatory tool to define adiposity, especially from professional medical organizations, is a testament to our knowledge gaps and our inaptitude in accepting that obesity is a disease involving abnormal fat, not simply the disease of an abnormally sized body.

Granted that we spend so much time and energy focusing on BMI, we mistakenly assume that all those with a bigger body size are unhealthy and those with a 'normal BMI' fall out of the risk bracket. And yes, it is true that if we focus on body fat composition and its function, we get much closer to the real problem: the percentage of abnormal body fat.

If the fat percentage largely determines healthy weight in our bodies, we immediately face an enormous challenge: How do we measure fat tissue percentage and its dysfunction in our body?

We can calculate body fat percentage in several ways. If you ever had your body composition assessed at a gym or by a dietitian, it was likely tested with calipers, which are small clamp-like devices that determine the amount of fat lying just below your skin. Calipers are most widely used due to their affordability and ease of use. However, they are not the most accurate indicator. Underwater weighing, the Bod Pod, DEXA (Dual-Energy X-ray Absorptiometry) scan and bioelectrical impedance analysis (BIA) are other methods of detecting body fat, which are less used due to their high cost. A DEXA bone densitometer can range from $17,000 to a massive $45,000 for a clinic, while a caliper costs $10 on Amazon.

Even if the total body fat is measured, no easy standardized tests are available to measure visceral and subcutaneous fat, body fluid status, muscle mass or bone mass. We need specialized equipment like DEXA scans and magnetic resonance imaging (MRIs) to quantify body fat and its distribution. Moreover, electronic body fat measurement technology is not readily available to everyone. One may argue that the use of wearable technology to test diverse biological and chemical compositions is rapidly on the rise. However, most wearable sensors are still ineffective for fat assessment.

Even if we measure the body's fat percentage, we are still far from assessing the percentage of fat that is dysfunctional. Currently, no appropriate test or technique is available to measure sick fat, which is the root cause of many adiposity-related problems.

Let's be clear on what we measure. When we read research papers stating that the 'prevalence of obesity increased from 12 per cent in 1991 to 18 per cent in 1998', it means that the percentage of people with a BMI greater than thirty in the population increased at that rate. This trend does not automatically translate to the percentage of sick fat in individuals.

So, What's the Solution Then?

To assess adiposopathy or dysfunctional fat, we need to shift from a weight-focused approach to a health-focused one. It has become clear that BMI alone is an inaccurate measure of adiposity, and measuring fat percentage is time-consuming and expensive. In this scenario, the best possible solution is to assess not one but a range of metabolic markers to better determine the degree of adiposity and its possible causes, and then arrive at solutions based on the disease's severity, not just on the person's size. 'Sick fat', which refers to adipose tissue (fat) that is behaving dysfunctionally or is associated with metabolic complications, can be measured using direct techniques such as body scans (computed tomography scans [CTs] or MRIs) and waist circumference. Other indirect methods such as blood tests that measure metabolic imbalances such as triglycerides, high-density lipoprotein (HDL) cholesterol, glucose, insulin and inflammatory markers like C-reactive protein (CRP) can give insights into the metabolic impact of one's body fat. Insulin sensitivity tests, such as the oral glucose tolerance test (OGTT) and the homeostatic model assessment for Insulin resistance (HOMA-IR) calculation, can offer insights into how one's adipose tissue is impacting metabolic function. Certain biomarkers are associated with adipose tissue dysfunction, including adipokines like leptin and adiponectin. When selecting a method to measure adiposity, it's essential to consider the accuracy, feasibility, cost and purpose (e.g., clinical practice, research, personal use).

To summarize how we have assessed and treated individuals with adiposity over the past half-century, the most honest thing to say is this: we have created a convenient way to measure a person's size and an imprecise way to measure abnormal fat tissue. Yes, we are still far from measuring the body's fat conveniently and accurately in a physician's office, but by acknowledging our knowledge gaps, moving towards technology-augmented research methods, and using better biomarkers to measure abnormal fat tissue, we have a better chance of addressing the problem.

A major part of the problem is due to the dichotomy between how obesity is studied by epidemiologists and what really happens in a body with excess and abnormal fat. BMI is a metric used by epidemiologists to measure trends among populations of different health conditions. To them, a higher BMI is *associated* with certain health problems, but in real life, it is abnormal fat that is the *cause* of obesity-related diseases.

Everything in this world exists on a spectrum. Fat is necessary, but we must guard against the development of sick fat. To date, we have cultivated an attitude of stigma and shame towards obese people in the absence of knowing a better way. We know now that obesity is not simply about appearance or a number on the weighing machine, but a disease that requires treatment—sensitive, empathetic, kind and professional treatment—the same as any other disease. The only way to do this is through education, not stigmatization, which continues to be a barrier to providing effective treatment to those in need.

At a Glance

❖ The biggest mistake in adiposity science is mistaking correlation with causation, i.e. linking signs and symptoms of a disease with the disease itself.

❖ The definition of adiposity doesn't say anything about body size or shape. However, the most widely accepted measure of adiposity in medical practice and society today is based only on body size and appearance.

- ❖ The greatest limitation of using body size as a surrogate to measure adiposity is that it is not suitable for assessing body fat.
- ❖ To compassionately and effectively address the disease of excess fat, we must reconsider BMI's role and its use as a screening tool than a diagnositic metric.
- ❖ The medical terminology should evolve from 'obesity' to 'adiposity', placing emphasis on fat content and composition rather than an individual's size.
- ❖ To define adiposity and treat it effectively, we need more than one tool.

* * *

Is Adiposity a Disease, an Illness or a Symptom?

'There's a huge difference between knowing the name of something and knowing something. We talk in fact-deficient, obfuscating generalities to cover up our lack of understanding.'

—Richard Feynman

In 1948, as the world emerged from the ashes of World War II and the WHO was taking its first steps, a bold proclamation was made: obesity was more than just a condition—it was a disease.[18] This audacious claim, however, seemed to vanish into the annals of time, overlooked for nearly fifty years. The 1980s brought renewed vigour from the WHO, armed with updated data, but the medical world continued to turn a blind eye. The tides finally shifted in 1998 when the NIH, the US government's bastion of medical research, took centre stage and unequivocally declared obesity a disease.

By June 2013, the American Medical Association house of delegates voted to acknowledge obesity as a disease that required treatment and preventive measures.[19] Numerous other professional medical organizations such as the Endocrine Society, the American College of Cardiology and the American Heart Association supported this idea. Many professional medical organizations around the world followed suit. Portugal recognized it as a chronic disease in 2004, Australia in 2018, Italy in 2019 and so on.

Designating a medical condition as a disease is not an easy task. The process involves teams of scientists, epidemiologists, clinicians and policymakers convening and delineating the rationale for elevating a medical condition to the status of a disease. For a medical condition to be declared a disease, it must fulfil three main criteria: (1) be heavily and unequivocally influenced by genetics, (2) have clear-cut signs and symptoms, and (3) demonstrate a proven mechanism of disease formation at the cellular level. In addition, it should cause distress and possibly death. Once a medical condition passes these rigorous criteria, the house of delegates in the American Medical Association (in the US or similar professional organizations in other countries) votes and releases a position statement.[20] The new disease is then included in medical education and finds a place in clinical practice. However, insurance providers (private or public) will allow payment coverage of the disease only when *they* acknowledge it as a disease that has adverse effects on an individual's health.

The terms 'disease' and 'illness' are often used interchangeably in our everyday life. However, these two concepts are distinct from one another. An illness is a subjective feeling of being sick, an experience that makes an individual visit a doctor. A disease is an underlying pathology in organs or tissues that can be examined and measured. High blood pressure, for instance, is categorized as a *disease* when blood pressure exceeds 140/90 mmHg, a threshold set by medical researchers and agreed upon by professional medical organizations. High blood pressure is not considered an *illness* by the individual because it is usually asymptomatic unless their blood pressure is high enough to cause discomfort or affect the individual's ability to function normally (like headache or dizziness).

Similarly, a person with early-stage cancer may not experience any feeling of illness while harbouring the disease. In contrast, a person with a fractured hip is immediately ill, instantly experiencing both a disease and an illness. A disease may be invisible and undetected; an illness is not.

According to Drew Leder's fascinating book *The Absent Body*, our bodies tend to self-conceal by quietly performing everyday processes and functions, meaning they are essentially 'absent'.[21] Our body parts stop being absent and become vividly present when certain biological processes cause them to go out of whack. Simply put: you don't feel your head until you have a headache. We don't feel our joints unless a step gives way to unstable ground. Similarly, a person with adiposity doesn't feel it unless it causes some discomfort, pain or debility; by this time, the disease has already set in.

Focusing solely on disease and illness in a health context neglects an essential facet of the human experience— suffering. Suffering is an intense experience that resonates both physically and mentally. It stands apart from its counterparts, disease and illness, as it impacts us on three fronts: physical, psychological and existential. Beyond its multidimensional impact, suffering spans a broad range of emotional distress. We can measure diseases using standardized biological parameters, and illnesses using graded scales and questionnaires. Suffering, however, is difficult to measure due to its complex, abstract presentation. Many factors can lead to suffering: inability to sleep, overeating, guilt, diminished self-esteem, and a lack of purpose and meaning. This immeasurable aspect of humans poses a challenge to the current dominant medical paradigm, where measured parameters drive most of the care and reimbursement decisions.

The problem is even more obvious when it comes to adiposity, a multidimensional disease. We don't have the faintest idea of measuring it in a way that encompasses all facets of the disease, let alone the suffering it causes.

Adiposity: Complex and Multifactorial

Back to our question: Is adiposity a disease, an illness or a symptom? It can be all three. It is a disease because it renders fat cells sick and triggers other physiological symptoms. It is an illness when individuals experience physical discomfort and suffer from its impact. It can also be a symptom of other medical conditions, such as Cushing's disease (caused by an excess steroid hormone called cortisol), Polycystic Ovarian Syndrome (PCOS) and eating disorders like binge eating. Adiposity could also be a symptom of emotional vulnerability, stress and lack of sleep. It could also be none of these, where the person is healthy but just living in a heavy body.

In the mid-1980s, health experts such as Professor Philip James, a world-renowned British scientist and one of the first people to identify the growing issue of obesity, noticed a baffling trend that people were getting fatter. The food industry promptly pointed out that individuals must be responsible for monitoring their calorie consumption, but even those who exercised and ate low-fat products were gaining weight. In 1966, only 1.2 per cent of men and 1.8 per cent of women had a BMI exceeding thirty (defined as obese).[22] The figures skyrocketed to 10.6 per cent for males and 14 per cent for women in 1989, but no one could see the link between the phenomenon of medical advancements and the ironically sick population. Meanwhile, by 2022, 42 per cent of the population was considered obese and this percentage continues to rise.[23]

Epidemiologists call this phenomenon an obesity epidemic. Charles Rosenberg, the author of *Explaining Epidemics*, notes that all epidemics end with a whimper, not with a bang—where the high disease incidence returns to its former levels.[24] An epidemic is an event in time, not a trend that moves perpetually without an end. The obesity phenomenon with its ever-rising rate, therefore, cannot be considered an epidemic.

We know, from many studies, that increased body fat was associated with increased morbidity and mortality in a population.[25] But we are still unsure about how to measure abnormal fat or what to call this phenomenon.

* * *

How Do Fat Cells Become Sick?

We have a love-hate relationship with our adipose tissue. Fat cells are second only to cancer cells as the most maligned cells in our body. Historically, it was assumed that fat was a passive stockpile of 'stuff' that served to insulate us from the cold. It was also a substance of cosmetic significance, smoothening wrinkles and helping lanky gentlemen appear 'full' in a suit. It wasn't until the early twentieth century that we learnt how fat cells store energy in the form of triglycerides. As research and development progressed in the latter half of the century, we learnt more about this previously elusive tissue. In the 1950s, scientists discovered that interrelated factors such as location, quantity and function of fat cells can have an impact on our metabolism.

According to the inaugural issue of the newly established *Journal of Lipid Research* in October 1959, adipose tissue was described as a 'metabolically active tissue containing most of the enzymes required to carry on reactions common to other mammalian tissues'.[26] This marked the commencement of lipid research, and new findings of how fat cells control metabolism began to emerge in the pages of the journal from its inception in 1959 until today.

Abnormal fat accumulation, as we now know, is about more than looks. Consider weight-loss surgery—people who were unsuccessful in losing weight naturally through dieting and exercising could drastically reduce their weight after the procedure. However, the benefits of this type of weight loss go beyond the number on the weighing scale. Numerous diseases such as diabetes, high blood pressure, excessive cholesterol, sleep apnea, heart disease and even mortality from some types of cancers, particularly colon and breast cancer, are now reduced by up to 60 per cent. The best outcome of all is an improvement in the quality of life.

Similar effects could be attained without going under the knife. A combination of controlled fasting and switching to a wholefood, plant-based diet is one such intervention. Although fasting is not for everyone, just like weight-loss surgery, it has been proven to successfully reverse many diseases, benefiting a vast number of people.

If one treatment or intervention (such as weight-loss surgery or fasting) can reverse many illnesses, it's a no-brainer to guess these diseases might have common pathways. When researchers studied the factors that led to overall health deterioration due to adiposity, they found one common pathway: chronic low-grade inflammation adversely affecting metabolism. Some research participants whose BMI was not in the overweight or obese range also experienced adverse inflammatory effects of abdominal fat, the most hormonally active component of total body fat. This illustrates that the harmful effects of abnormal fat cells can affect anyone, regardless of the person's size.

To fully comprehend how inflammation results in diseases due to metabolic dysfunction, we need to understand the role of fat in overall health, especially in the development of diseases that can cause debility or shorten our lifespan. This knowledge gap is one of the major causes for the needless shaming heavy people have to go through, because we fail to recognize that their adiposity is due to the abnormal fat cells wreaking havoc on their overall health.

What Exactly Is Fat and What Does It Do?

Metabolism refers to the sum total of all the chemical reactions in a living cell that convert food energy into kinetic energy used for bodily functions. It is how the body expends energy at rest and during activity.

You are probably familiar with the role of carbohydrates and proteins in your metabolic function. Carbohydrates provide quick energy, and proteins facilitate enzyme activities and structure, growth and maintenance of cells and tissues. However, the role of fat in our metabolism is often poorly understood. Our understanding of adiposity is incomplete if we do not understand the essential role of fat in overall metabolism.

Generally speaking, eating a meal creates a positive energy balance in our bodies. During times without energy intake, like during sleep or fasting, our bodies dip into the available energy stores and enter into a negative energy balance. In short, energy storage after feeding and energy expenditure during fasting are like the yin and yang of our physiology.

Fat Cell and Its Function

Fats are high energy-producing molecules stored in clusters of compounds called triacylglycerols, commonly known as triglycerides. A fat cell or adipocyte is simply a droplet of the fat reservoir, i.e. triacylglycerol, swaddled in a slimy layer with a nucleus at the top. It is the only cell in our body where a stockpile of energy takes up 90 per cent of the cytoplasm or internal space.

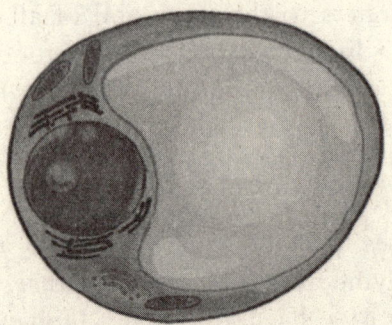

Figure 2.1: A fat cell under a microscope appears as a large, clear bubble filled with lipid, pushing the nucleus and other organelles to its periphery

A young adult male weighing 70 kg has about 15–20 kg of fat storage (the actual quantity varies widely depending on age, gender, ethnicity and many other factors).

The body obtains fats through two primary means: the first is directly from food and the second is by converting the carbohydrates consumed. The body converts the excess carbohydrates into fatty acids through complex chemical reactions, mainly in the liver and adipose tissue. Interestingly, carbs and fat conversion is usually a one-way street; ingested carbs are converted to fats for storage. The reverse is possible but rarely happens. The human body rarely converts fats into carbs because it involves a convoluted and cumbersome process. Carbons from fat breakdowns are funnelled through uncommon chemical pathways and ultimately make their way into glycogen (the storage form of sugar) production, which are further broken down to glucose. The entire roundabout process uses lots of energy and is hence an unrewarding exercise for the cell except in extreme starvation.

On the other hand, fat genesis is gold for the body because each gram of fat can provide more than twice the energy supplied by proteins or carbohydrates. Because of its high energy efficiency, the body goes to extreme lengths to capture every bit of fat from foods consumed and store them. For instance, when you eat a peanut butter sandwich, the first thing your body does is reduce the triglycerides in the peanut butter into fatty acids, which then enter the tiny intestinal cells (called enterocytes), where they are reassembled into new triglycerides. Each tiny particle then attaches itself to a protein and cholesterol molecule to form a bigger particle called chylomicron. These chylomicron clusters are then released into the blood to circulate. They are our body's way of ferrying the triglycerides into our tissues for energy production or to store them as fat for further use.

When the energy expenditure exceeds what's immediately available for the body, these stored triacylglycerols are released from the fat cells, a process referred to as fat breakdown. The triacylglycerols break away from the glycerol molecule, leaving 'free fatty acids' (FFA). These are then released into the blood and transported to other tissues that need energy, usually muscle cells.

These FFAs are further broken down once they reach the target muscle cells that demand energy. Here, a crucial enzyme called LPL, or lipoprotein lipase, admits our FFAs to the mitochondria, the powerhouse of a cell. The final products of fat metabolism are then expertly processed, first through a breakdown process known as beta oxidation. This is where fatty acids are cleaved and then channelled through a multistep process known as the citric acid cycle to release energy that can be stored in the form of Adenosine triphosphate (ATP). ATP is the ultimate molecule that absorbs chemical energy from the breakdown of food molecules and releases it to fuel other cellular processes.

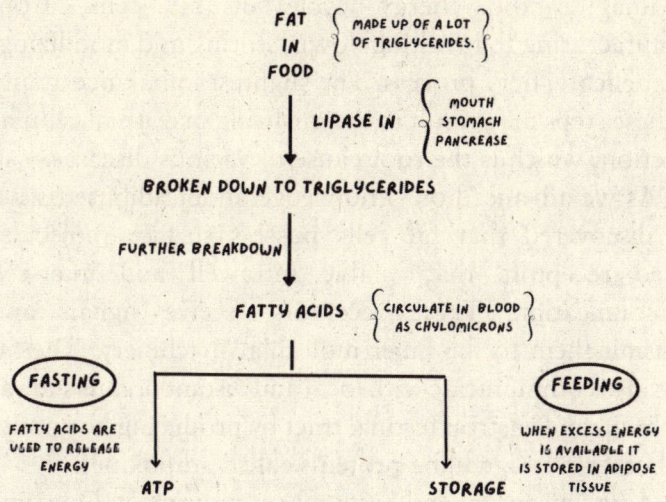

Figure 2.2: The fat breakdown process

Excess Adipose Tissue Is Not Just about Quantity but Has More to Do with the Quality of Fat Tissue

The human body has approximately 600 types of fats that we know of.[27] Did you know that triglycerides, cholesterol and essential fatty acids have many subtypes? These cell types are ubiquitous in our bodies. The functions of our body fats include storing energy, behaving as messengers, allowing cells to send and receive information, and helping proteins function. In short, fats protect all vital organs involved in growth, immunity and reproduction, and serve as metabolic defenders for all organs throughout their lifespan.

Imagine the energy cycle of fat cells, from manufacturing to breaking down, storing and mobilizing, as a delicate, fiery process. The slightest imbalance at any of these steps may result in the misfiring of normal cellular function, which is the root cause of various diseases.

As we advanced our knowledge about adipose tissue, we discovered that fat cells possess surface molecules called receptors that enable intra-cell and inter-cell communication. These receptors receive signals and transmit them to the inner molecular machinery. The fat cells also communicate with local and distant organs such as the brain and gastrointestinal tract by producing hormones and other cell-signalling proteins called adipokines.

Adipo means fat and *kinos* means movement. One such adipokine called *leptin* increases in tandem with the number of fat cells. The discovery of leptin in 1994 revealed that fat cells could essentially 'talk' to the brain about energy storage in the body and its nutritional status. Derived from the Greek root *leptos*, which means thin, leptin informs the brain when the body has enough stored fat, which signals the body to curb appetite and burn calories normally.

What's more intriguing is that many tissues in our body, like muscle and beta cells of the pancreas (where insulin is produced), have specific receptors on their cells that can recognize leptin molecules. This arrangement allows leptin to control the various peripheral tissues. The primary role of leptin is to convey the energy status to the organs and tissues in our body. Consequently, the body produces more leptin during a fat surplus and reduces it during a fat deficit. What makes this hormone even more exciting (or scary) is its direct effects on reproductive organs like the ovaries and testes. Animal experiments show that excess leptin (seen in states of excess fat stores) accelerates puberty in normal female mice and hypogonadism (reduced reproductive hormone production) in male subjects. In addition, leptin affects bone development, wound healing and immune function. This modus operandi of fat tissue is similar to the workings of endocrine organs such as the thyroid or adrenals.

Not all hormones produced by fat cells are harmful. Interestingly, leptin was discovered roughly at the same time as another hormone, which has opposite effects. Adiponectin, a hormone with far-reaching effects, also produced in the fat cell was discovered in 1995. It is anti-diabetic, anti-inflammatory and anti-atherogenic (lessens the formation of fatty plaques in the arteries).

Fat tissue is now firmly recognized as a metabolically active endocrine organ and a crucial player in energy homeostasis after the discovery of hormones like leptin and adiponectin that facilitate energy balance.

* * *

The body has two main types of fat tissue used to store energy—white and brown. The fat cells in these tissues behave differently based on their characteristics and location, acting regiospecifically. For example, white fat is found under the skin, mostly in the abdomen, thighs and buttocks. In moderate amounts, this fat is helpful— it stores energy and secretes hormones to regulate our impulse to eat. Brown fat, on the other hand, is primarily used in heat regulation, especially in babies. It is located in the upper back, neck and shoulders.

By studying the origins of these tissues, we learn a lot about their functions. Brown adipose tissue's forerunners are related to myocytes (muscle cells). A brown fat cell or brown adipose tissue is very dense in mitochondria, the cellular powerhouse of energy, which gives it its colour. It has a unique mechanism where the energy within brown fat cells is utilized to generate heat. In contrast, white adipose tissue stores energy as triglycerides and releases it as fatty acids. White fat cells are distinguished by their friendly metabolic activity.

Together, the white and brown adipose tissue coordinate as an active, metabolic 'organ', performing a multitude of functions throughout the entire body.

How Normal Fat Cells Become Sick

To appreciate why the benevolent adipose tissue turns against its host, we must first understand *what* makes fat cells 'sick' and examine *how* a normal fat cell becomes precarious. This knowledge is crucial to address the diseases that sick fat cells mercilessly provoke.

Normal adipose tissue becomes ill under two broad circumstances—the first is energy surplus. When we consume more food than the body requires to carry out all of its metabolic activities, the energy surplus creates an excessive accumulation of fat and triggers a gradual deterioration in adipose tissue health. When the body experiences a constant surplus of energy, it causes the fat cells to enlarge. This process is called hypertrophy, the body's natural response to the storage of excess energy. A normal fat cell expands like a balloon until it reaches its limit, during which it undergoes biochemical modifications.

The second and most important stimuli are outside disruptors that are consumed daily. These non-energy substances make adipose tissue sick as they accumulate in these cells. Their list is expansive and includes fructose, refined grains, uric acid, food preservatives, colouring agents, taste-enhancing additives and certain environmental pollutants. These endocrine disruptors are ubiquitous in plastic products, synthetic chemicals in fragrances, household chemicals, detergents, pesticides, etc.

Until 2008, most people believed that our bodies maintain a constant amount of fat cells under typical circumstances. Adiposity research revealed that excess calorie intake causes not just an expansion of the fat cell but also the multiplication of fat cells, a condition known as hyperplasia.

The metabolic demands of these enlarged fat cells soon exceed the nourishment their blood supply can provide, leading to an imbalance between demand and supply. This results in hypoxia, a condition where fat cells lacking adequate oxygen supply die prematurely. In these low oxygen conditions, the initial casualties are the cell's intracellular structures: the mitochondria, which serve as the cell's powerhouses, and the endoplasmic reticulum, a fine network of interconnected tubes inside the cell. As these structures deteriorate, they progressively lose functionality.

Fat cells can go rogue even in a non-obese state, as in the case of someone with a normal BMI but high visceral (or abdominal) fat mass. The pathway to disease causation is the same regardless of what stimuli turn good fat sick—inflammation. Normally, inflammation occurs due to increased blood flow, increased permeability of blood vessels, and the migration of fluid, proteins and white blood cells to the site of the tissue damage. It occurs due to physical trauma like a burn, cut or bruise, or a viral, bacterial or fungal infection. Inflammation is a natural response that occurs when such damage is done to living tissues and its purpose is to fight the threat to the immune system. Once the threat has passed, the inflammation subsides. But when that inflammation becomes chronic and doesn't subside after its intended task is over, it becomes a problem. Chronic inflammation brings a long list of complications, including arthritis, asthma, atherosclerosis, blindness, cancer, diabetes and, quite possibly, even mental illnesses.

Earlier, we considered all fat to be 'bad', but now we understand that normal fat and sick fat are two vastly different entities. While fat is naturally occurring and crucial to the metabolism of the body, sick fat is the product of abnormal conditions. It begins when fat cells expand superfluously and interfere with normal fat metabolism. As the number and size of fat cells within the body grow, the inflammatory effect within the tissues also multiplies. A ripple effect carries this harm to the various organs throughout our body, resulting in a condition known as adiposopathy (adipose-opathy), an anatomical and functional adipocyte dysfunction.

The Genesis of Inflammation within the Sick Fat Cells

In response to the stress within the sick fat cells, a type of white blood cell called macrophages infiltrates the adipocytes and starts a cascade of inflammation.

Macrophages are born out of a particular type of white blood cells called monocytes, and are responsible for locating and devouring microbes like bacteria, viruses, fungi and parasites. Even though foreign microbes do not invade the fat cells, the body recognizes the cellular stress as a threat and dispatches macrophages to the expanding fat tissues.

The inflammatory effects of fat tissue macrophages are mediated through specific chemicals called cytokines (specifically IL6 and TNF-α). Unfortunately, the damage caused due to inflammation doesn't stop there. They also contribute to the recruitment of additional macrophages by secreting other chemicals like chemokines or chemoattractant cytokines (MCP-1 and MIP-1α).

MCP stands for Monocyte Chemoattractant Protein, a special type of protein released by fat cells which attracts monocytes. MIP, Macrophage Inflammatory Protein, is another inflammatory protein secreted by fat cells. Usually, the elevation of chemokines is seen in states of inflammation like infections and autoimmune diseases. Since obese individuals have significantly more of these inflammatory proteins, scientists hypothesize that these chemokines play an essential role in developing metabolic complications in people with adiposity.

When infiltrated by macrophages, fat cells, especially visceral fat, become 'metabolically active' to create and sustain a state of low-grade chronic inflammation due to an overexcited immune system. This hypothesis explains the following cascade of events: first, macrophages are recruited to adipose tissue, then the macrophage–

adipocyte interactions result in an inflammatory cascade that contributes to adiposity-related pathophysiological conditions like insulin resistance, dyslipidemia, diabetes, cardiovascular disease, cancers, autoimmune diseases and others.

How Sick Fat Cells Cause Diseases

No single organ or organ system is unaffected by adiposopathy. From pulmonary diseases to liver diseases, gynaecological abnormalities and strokes, most of our physiology is affected. Emerging research also suggests a correlation between excess body fat and an *increased risk* of several cancers, including colorectal, postmenopausal breast, uterine, oesophageal, kidney and pancreatic. In most cases, it is due to the chronic low-level inflammation-induced damage to our DNA over time.

We can examine the link between adiposopathy and related diseases through mechanical, functional and direct effects of abnormal fat cells.

> Adiposity means excess fat. Adiposopathy is the presence of dysfunctional fat tissue (the 'sick fat')

Mechanical Effects

The mechanical properties of normal tissues are usually the first to be altered by excess fat accumulation. For instance, we know that overweight individuals are more likely to have conditions such as acid reflux and gall bladder problems than normal-weight individuals. The chronic inflammation due to gastroesophageal reflux disease leads to a precancerous condition called Barrett's oesophagus, a precursor to oesophageal cancer. We also know that these individuals are at a high risk of gallstone formation and chronic gall bladder inflammation, a vital risk factor for gall bladder cancer.

Excess fat accumulation often impacts the lungs, leading to structural changes in the airways and subsequent respiratory problems. Issues such as impaired gas exchange, heightened airway resistance, diminished lung volume and weakened muscle strength can enhance vulnerability to conditions like pulmonary hypertension or high lung pressures. Over time, this can strain the heart, potentially resulting in heart failure. Moreover, these airway alterations may hinder recovery in patients with lung infections.

Functional Effects

High blood pressure, also known as hypertension, adversely affects almost every organ in the body, with strokes being the most dangerous, and heart and kidney diseases trailing behind.

Since their discovery in 1898, the Renin–Angiotensin System (RAS) protein family has been implicated in increasing vascular tone, sodium and water retention, and stimulating the secretion of stress hormones from adrenals. The net result is higher blood pressure. For a long time, since the 1930s, the liver and kidneys were the only two organs thought to be involved in angiotensin and its family of hormones.

However, in the late 1980s, we discovered that the RAS protein is also expressed in the fat cells and plays a vital role in regulating blood pressure. The higher the fat mass, the higher the RAS proteins and the blood pressure. When scientists made research participants lose excess fat through fasting, it resulted in a decreased expression of RAS proteins on the fat cells, which correlated with a lowered (improved) blood pressure. The RAS expression on fat cells and blood pressure increased when the participants were fed in excess. This effect was observed in both genders. Researchers believe that the fat tissue RAS is a potential link between high blood pressure and adiposopathy. Besides hormone-mediated effects, fat tissue around the artery wall restricts its elasticity, causing high blood pressure. Apart from the RAS protein-mediated blood pressure effects, excess fat tissue causes hypertension through hyperaldosteronism or high aldosterone (a salt regulating hormone) levels from an increase in an enzyme called aldosterone synthase in the adipocyte. Decrease in adipocytes through weight loss lowers aldosterone levels and hence lowers blood pressure.

For years, we understood that there was a link between adiposopathy and high blood pressure but didn't know the reason. We were aware that increased weight often meant higher blood pressure. Now, we've learnt that unhealthy fat tissue can lead to hypertension because of its hormonal and mechanical impacts. Essentially, high blood pressure can be seen as a sign of chronic inflammation from unhealthy fat and recent studies back this up.

Adiposity leads to hypertension via RAS and aldosterone-driven pathways. Moreover, fat build-up in and around the kidney, often referred to as fatty kidney disease, plays a role in exacerbating chronic kidney disease. Shedding this harmful excess fat is key to mitigating the damage or decelerating the advancement of kidney deterioration.

Direct Effects

Finally, we have the dominant culprit behind many chronic diseases—insulin resistance. This condition is associated with type 2 diabetes mellitus, polycystic ovarian diseases, fatty liver disease, depression, early-onset dementia and many cancers.

Excess fatty acids in the bloodstream enter the muscle cells, generating breakdown products called *intramyocellular lipids*. These tiny fat globules within the muscle cells are the primary disruptors of the insulin-signalling mechanism, causing the cells to be resistant to insulin. As a result, the glucose levels in the blood continue rising uncontrollably. Consequently, insulin resistance stimulates the pancreas to produce more insulin until it burns out and stops entirely. The result is type 2 diabetes, a *symptom* of fat cell dysfunction.

Insulin is also involved in satiety. When cells become resistant to insulin, satiation is diminished. We crave instant energy-generating foods like refined carbs, which leads to further adiposity and the vicious spiral continues.

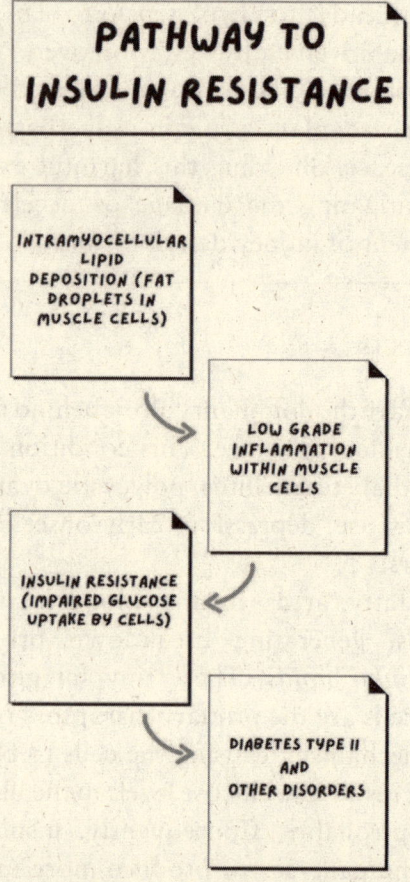

Figure 2.3: Pathway to Insulin Resistance

Cancers Due to Adiposity

Decades ago, medical scientists discovered that conditions such as ulcerative colitis and hepatitis significantly increase the likelihood of colon and liver cancers. Through its chronic inflammatory effects, we now know that adiposity is responsible for developing many gastrointestinal malignancies, including pancreatic, colon, liver, oesophagus, gastric and gall bladder cancers. Furthermore, since abnormal fat accumulation increases blood insulin levels and insulin-like growth factors, this may promote the development of colon, kidney, prostate and endometrial cancers.

Adiposopathy has long been known to raise the risk of cancer in the female reproductive tract, as evidenced by an article published in the *American Journal of Clinical Nutritionists* in 1987 titled 'Adipose Tissue as a Source of Hormones'.[28] Unfortunately, this is still a little-known reality among many medical professionals. Most practising clinicians are unaware that adipose tissue produces up to 100 per cent of all circulating oestrogen in postmenopausal women. The greater your fat mass, the higher the oestrogen levels in your body, which raises the risk of breast cancer in postmenopausal women. Adiposity not only increases the risk but often leads to poor prognosis in people who are affected by breast cancer.

Sick fat is responsible for all stages of cancer, from cancer formation to progression to relapse. While sick fat is linked to the increased aggressiveness of many types of cancers, it can also make cancer cells resistant to treatment.

Anything that reduces adiposopathy reduces chronic low-grade inflammation as well.

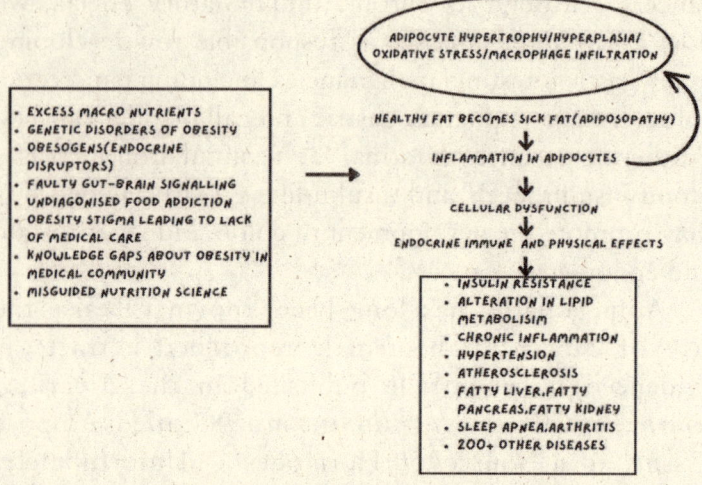

Figure 2.4: Obesity and Inflammation

Despite the growing knowledge on how adiposopathy may contribute to various cancers, this problem is still not taken seriously in many cancer clinics. Why? Given that almost all of the data from these cancer–adiposopathy studies comes from observational studies, some argue that correlation is not causation. Despite the limitations of the study designs, medical scientists were able to ascertain that a higher amount of abnormal body fat is indeed associated with an increased risk of several cancers. Nevertheless, we have yet to establish a distinct causal relationship between cancer and sick fat.

> Not only is sick fat linked to increased aggressiveness of many types of cancers, but it can also make cancer cells resistant to treatment.

Ultimately, what matters with sick fat are the diseases it generates. At each stage of a disease, i.e. primary, secondary or tertiary prevention of adiposopathy, all scientific organizations emphasize one particular recommendation: healthy lifestyle changes. This involves reduced calories, healthy meal plans, physical activity and education. The solution seems straightforward—change your lifestyle to become leaner. However, it is easier said than done. You will face many barriers in achieving this, including the very science that recommends this pathway. The subsequent chapters expose different obstacles to recognizing and treating the problem of adiposopathy.

At a Glance

❖ Adiposopathy is consistently associated with chronic low-grade inflammation of adipose tissue.

❖ Sick fat is associated with mechanical and functional alterations of tissues.

❖ Despite the growing knowledge about how adiposopathy may cause different types of cancers, this problem is still not taken seriously in cancer clinics as we have yet to establish a causal relationship between cancer and dysfunctional fat.

3

Wired for Regaining Weight

Inspirational weight-loss stories portrayed in reality shows like *The Biggest Loser,* and the 'before' and 'after' images featured in magazines are deceptive. They don't reveal the big picture. As many as 90 per cent of people who have lost considerable weight will gain it back in one to five years, regardless of the method used.[1] It is tempting to see this as a moral failing of the individual. In this scenario, rather than shaming or, even worse, sympathizing with the person who struggles to maintain a healthy weight, the most logical thing to do is to ask the right questions: *what makes our body regain excess weight every time we try to lose it and what can we do about it?*

Set Point Theory

Numerous theories were proposed to explain our body's perpetual drive to regain its lost weight. One dominant theory explaining this phenomenon is the set point theory. According to this theory, our body has a 'set point', a weight at which it naturally tends to return to. The set point theory actually applies to several parameters in our innards and is not exclusive to body weight. Consider body temperature. Our core temperature is maintained at around 36.5–37.5 °C. This is tightly regulated by various 'thermostats' spread throughout our body. If the hypothalamus in our brain detects changes in the core temperature, it will send signals to the peripheral tissues to increase sweating or shivering, or moderate our body temperature through other mechanisms.[2] Similarly, our body has numerous mechanisms to tightly control its blood pressure, blood sugar, blood pH and electrolytes (like sodium, potassium, calcium, etc.) within a certain range for optimal functioning of its organs.

Our set point weight is orchestrated by multiple biological feedback control mechanisms coordinated between the central nervous system and peripheral tissues. Unfortunately, this regulation is asymmetric, where our body is more responsive to weight loss than weight gain.[3] Tragically, our weight can increase without limit. We will burn more of our energy sources if we fast or expend lots of energy through high-intensity workouts, but the converse is not true; consuming more calories does not mean we will expend more of our energy reserves.

When you decrease calorie intake by eating sparingly, the body adjusts by slowing down its metabolism, a process known as adaptive thermogenesis. This ingenious metabolic compensation aims to reserve stored fats for any future energy expenditure. This preservation strategy allows even underweight people to function physiologically despite adopting an unbelievably low-calorie diet. This phenomenon also explains why underweight individuals tend to feel cold most of the time—because the body spends less energy warming itself to conserve energy. Adaptive thermogenesis is lifesaving during a legitimate famine.[4] In instances of food scarcity, the body will express gratitude for this survival mechanism. Still, it is also inevitably more frustrating and depressing when the body actively resists one's effort to lose weight.

Besides slowing down your metabolism when you cut back on calories, your mind and body also fight to increase appetite, compelling you to eat. The result is a rapid weight rebound the moment you return to a regular diet. This yo-yoing is frequently observed in those who follow the ketogenic (minimal carb, high fat) diet, which can be very effective in weight loss. However, the minute they discontinue this diet, they gradually regain all the lost weight.[5]

> Your body has a 'set point', a weight at which it naturally tends to return to.

On top of the body's recoiling tendency to regain lost weight, it is also possible that a person will gain weight *even* if they exercise regularly. Physical training helps improve the strength and efficiency of your heart, lungs and muscles. While this is priceless if you are trying to improve your heart–lung function, it causes sheer frustration in the long run if you are trying to lose weight. With improved muscle efficiency, you might notice your morning jog getting easier over time, which seems like a good thing, but it also means you are burning less energy than before to do the same intensity of exercise—you won't be burning as many calories as you were before unless you start jogging a little faster or increase the distance jogged.

Feast and Famine—Minus the Famine

To survive the famine in the earlier days, our ancestors had to fast (actually, starve) intermittently, so their bodies could gradually evolve to live and function normally in such conditions. Society has evolved and so have our social conditions. Our bodies, however, have not evolved as rapidly. When you reduce your food intake, your body's evolutionary instinct kicks in, assuming that you are in a state of famine.

Our hunter–gatherer forefathers survived the days when food was scarce. Their bodies were designed to preserve internal balance and utilize energy as efficiently as possible despite a low caloric intake. Our ancestors certainly didn't eat three meals and two snacks a day—they were uncertain about when their next meal would come. They ate only when food was available. The body saved the surplus energy from those precious meals for future activities that involved high energy expenditure, such as hunting, gathering, evading predators and caring for weaker members of the tribe. Due to this adaptation, their metabolism slowed down during a sudden decline in their caloric intake to ration out the energy for as long as possible, so that they could continue their activities normally.

For 3,00,000 years, human survival depended on the tight balance between energy consumption and expenditure. Our bodies adapted to store energy in the form of fats while sporting a physique of leanness with manoeuvrability to aid in escaping predators. The human species survived and thrived thanks to our ability to store and metabolize fats efficiently.

Humans would have been extinct by now if our metabolism was not so adaptable and flexible. A man weighing 75 kg typically has over 1,00,000 kcal of energy stored in the form of fats in his body. Assuming this man is around thirty-five years old and about 5' 9", his basic metabolic rate (BMR) is 1755 calories a day. That means his body burns 1755 calories a day for its basic metabolic functions, such as breathing, circulating blood and executing various cellular processes. Even at 2000 calories, the reasonably modest fat reserves mean that a 75-kg man could theoretically survive on water alone for up to fifty days, provided accidents, suicide or infections don't kill him first.

We evolved into a successful species by being active and agile in the hunting grounds, chasing fast-moving prey and fleeing from swift predators. A turning point for our species was around 12,000 years ago when our ancestors gave up their nomadic, hunter–gatherer lives, and shifted to living in settlements, building fixed communities, planting crops and domesticating livestock. The advent of agriculture marked the first semblance of food reliability that humanity had ever known.

As people became more adept at farming, food sources became more accessible and populations began to boom. During the Industrial Revolution (1760–1910), the introduction of farm machinery made food supplies even more abundant than before while also displacing a huge number of workers in the agricultural sector. Technological advances that began in the late nineteenth century ultimately led to the mass production of food in large factories, providing a constant supply of food that we have at our fingertips today.

Today's world is vastly different from that of our hunter–gatherer ancestors and our genes are not yet prepared to face the current food environment. The majority of people in developed countries do not face food supply uncertainty and starvation is as unlikely as being mauled by a sabre-toothed tiger. We are faced with a completely different problem, one which our ancestors would have never expected in their wildest dreams— overnutrition.

The mechanism that helped humans dominate the world is now contributing to adiposity-related illnesses. Your body constantly stockpiles energy in the form of fats for a famine that will never come.

Weight Loss, Hormones and the Brain

Your body's energy reserves are under tight neuro-hormonal control. Specific areas in your brain orchestrate food cravings, such as the hypothalamus which is located at the base of the brain. Its complex positive and negative feedback loops appetite control and hunger sensations. Compulsive feelings and cravings for food, especially those associated with reward and pleasure, are regulated by the hypothalamus. When your brain detects a decreased caloric intake, the hypothalamus releases hormones such as neuropeptide Y (NPY)[6] and glucocorticoids (a stress hormone). Together, these hormones make it difficult to resist compulsive eating during times of caloric restrictions, aka restrictive dieting or fasting. The result is weight regain and fat accumulation.

Leptin is another hormone related to feelings of hunger and satiety.[7] It is a chemical derived from fat cells which sends signals to the brain (specifically the hypothalamus) when you are satiated and breaks down the adipose tissue. It also informs the brain about the levels of or changes in fat mass so that the brain can send appropriate signals to modulate energy intake and expenditure.

Leptin-mediated fat regulation is asymmetric, similar to set point theory. This hormone defends your body against fat loss, but it does not protect your body against fat regain; leptin shows its prowess only when you lose weight. When fat cells shrink upon losing weight, less leptin is produced, which signals the brain to conserve energy, thereby triggering the metabolism to burn fewer calories and minimize weight loss.

Another part of the brain that plays a role in food regulation is the amygdala, where the reward centre resides.[8] Ever heard the saying, 'hunger is the best spice'? When you're hungry, the amygdala suggests that everything tastes better, prompting you to eat. As you become full, this effect diminishes, signalling that you've consumed enough. Those who strongly react to food cues in the amygdala are more prone to regaining weight after shedding it. They often don't feel content, even after eating sufficiently. The brain's reward centres can undermine their weight maintenance efforts. Even if leptin signals fullness, the area of the brain responsible for food restraint becomes less responsive after weight loss. This makes maintaining weight (and preserving willpower) even tougher than the initial weight-loss process.

This leptin and neuropeptide Y-mediated response explains why it is easier to gain and keep weight than lose it. After a diet restriction, the drive to overeat seeks to restore the fat reserves to their initial state. It is beyond just a mental response to the weeks of deprivation—it is a biological call demanding the body to replenish the fat reserves.

Simply put, when you cut down on calories, specific changes occur in your body's hormones and brain chemistry.[9] These changes cause your metabolism to fight against weight loss and attempt to recover the lost fat, making the calorie-counting method of dieting challenging. It's as if nature has crafted a challenging obstacle course on our path to weight loss.

Gut Microbiome[10]

During her appointment with her dietician, Marcia, a fifty-five-year-old Brazilian woman, complained discontentedly that she and her husband practically ate the same meal every day. Despite consuming far more goodies than her and exercising rarely, he maintained a healthy weight. This irony made her resentful and she couldn't wrap her head around it.

The hundreds of microbial species crowding her gut, fighting to dominate it, are part of the answer. The gut microbiome, a fundamental component of the colon's landscape, has significantly impacted human health. Besides the fact that the gut bacteria outnumber the total number of human cells, it's interesting to note that the microbe's genome also cross-talks with its host's (i.e. your) genome and alters it, either positively or negatively.[11] An adiposogenic diet, a diet high in fat and sugar, primes the microbiome long before the development of adiposity.

Scientists are still working to understand the mechanism behind this, but what we know so far is already mind-blowing. The gut microbiome is a complex ecosystem with colonies of healthy and bad bacteria strewn all over the intestine.

The dominant bacterial colonies in the gut ecosystem determine the microbiome's characteristics. *Firmicutes* and *Bacteroides* are the two most common gut bacteria, accounting for 92 per cent of the gut flora.[12] Whether a person is lean or obese depends on the ratio of these two bacteria. An individual with a higher level of Bacteroides tends to be leaner than one with a higher Firmicutes load.

Imagine that you ate oatmeal for breakfast and cornmeal for lunch. They both contain dietary fibre, often known as indigestible polysaccharides. The friendly bacteria help extract energy from indigestible polysaccharide-rich meals. The colon's microbiome is responsible for breaking down the complex polysaccharides since our bodies lack specific enzymes needed to break them down. Besides breaking down the complex polysaccharides, gut bacteria can also change their microbial species to adapt to the diet we eat. These microbes break down the complex polysaccharides in our diet into simpler monosaccharides and fatty acids, which are quickly absorbed by the gut and transported to the liver to manufacture triglycerides, a type of fat in the blood.

Assuming you and your partner lead similar lifestyles and share a comparable diet, one might struggle with weight while the other remains unaffected. You could have gut microbes that draw more energy from food, whereas your partner's microbiome might extract less. This means that even when eating the same meals and engaging in the same activities, one of you might gain weight while the other doesn't. The efficiency with which one's gut microbes extract energy from food can play a significant role in weight differences, potentially making weight loss more challenging for some than for others.

Microbial community composition in our gut is determined incredibly early in our lives, starting at birth and reaching its maturity by the age of three. On a positive note, our dietary environment can also play a major role in altering that bacterial composition. Research conducted by Peter J. Turnbaugh and his team in 2009 showed that one who adopts a Western diet, which is high in animal fat, had a significantly lower proportion of Bacteroides and a higher proportion of Firmicutes. On the other hand, those who follow a diet high in fibre, plants, fruits and legumes will have much higher proportions of Bacteroides and lower proportions of Firmicutes.[13] This latter composition is more favourable for maintaining a healthy weight.

Since 2009, researchers have conducted many more experiments to explore how food consumption alters the composition of bacteria in the gut and how this alteration influences an individual's metabolism, either positively or negatively. Furthermore, many more bacteria were identified that influence the host's metabolism.[14]

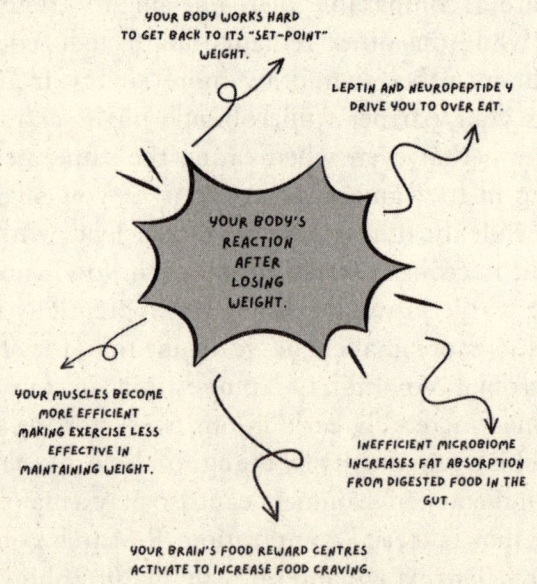

Figure 3.1: What Happens to Your Body After You Lose Weight?

Experts Take On What We Should Actually Do

Contrary to popular belief, regaining weight after successfully losing it is not due to lack of willpower. Environmental, biochemical and genetic variables all contribute to the relentlessness of the yo-yo effect.

Yes, it's a struggle. Your body wants to defend its weight.[15] Researchers argue that simply resisting the urge to eat through sheer willpower may not work. It is also unhelpful to eat loads of low-calorie veggies to fool your mind and convince yourself that you are full. If it is unsustainable to fight the hunger and hope that the feeling will eventually disappear, what other methods could work?

The rule of thumb is to genuinely lower your set point so that losing weight and keeping it off is attainable. You also need to recognize and accept that losing weight is not a linear process. As human beings, we will gain weight and lose some throughout our lives. This fluctuation is normal. Given that multiple factors determine our weight, we need a variety of solutions, too; implementing only one technique on its own does not help. We do not have a single one-size-fits-all solution and what works for one person may not work for another.

Medical experts suggest that it is better to work alongside your physiology instead of against it.[16] Four strategies have been shown to lower the set point weight and maintain it for a long time. They are:

1. The 10 per cent solution
2. Time-restricted eating

3. Develop a healthy microbiome
4. Reduce adiposogens (adiposity generators)

The 10 Per Cent Solution[17]

Scientific research supports losing no more than 10 per cent of your body weight at a time. You may start with 5 per cent as your initial target and work your way up. It turns out that 10 per cent is the amount of weight you can lose before your body starts to counter it. Numerous clinical studies have confirmed this phenomenon. Of course, it is possible to lose more than 10 per cent at one go but only a small percentage of people sustain that loss.

You can consider changing your diet and exercise routine every six months to sustain your weight loss and maintain the newly attained lighter weight or even drop another 10 per cent. By re-evaluating your diet and lifestyle from time to time (for instance, every six months), you effectively lower your body's set point. Even if you do not maintain your new lower weight for good, making slight, incremental modifications to your everyday choices significantly increases your chances of success. It's a technique that has been proven to bypass the starvation response to regain prior levels of fats, retrain the amygdala's reaction to palatable food cues and boost Bacteroides levels in the gut microbiome.

This approach has also been proven to re-establish a new set point weight. Sometimes, this slows down your weight-loss curve, but in the long run, you are providing time for your brain to catch up with what the body is doing, giving it a chance to work for you rather than against you.

Time-Restricted Eating (TRE)[18]

Intermittent fasting has become increasingly popular among both health experts and the general public, offering a variety of approaches. Alternate-day fasting, alternate-day modified fasting, 5:2 diet, fasting-mimicking diet and time-restricted eating are the most commonly researched forms of intermittent fasting. It's an approach focusing on *when* you eat rather than *what* you eat.

Our bodies are governed by the circadian rhythm—physical, mental and behavioural changes that follow a twenty-four-hour cycle. This natural process affects all living beings, including animals, plants and even microbes. For example, our natural human tendency to sleep at night and wake during the day is part of our circadian rhythm. Hence, the name 'circa' meaning about and 'dian' meaning day. Our metabolism naturally follows our hormones as they fluctuate in accordance with our circadian rhythm.

When it comes to energy utilization, our body first uses the readily available carbs from the food we consume before tapping into its reserves and burning the fat for energy. Intermittent fasting intentionally restricts food for a prolonged period to mobilize the stored fat. This is accomplished by picking a specific feeding and fasting window in a twenty-four-hour cycle.

Intermittent fasting enables our body to repair and regenerate without interference. In this context, the most common interference to this process is frequent snacking. Fasting for eighteen hours or more activates cellular self-repair pathways. Autophagy or cellular self-cleaning process, is the body's way of keeping our cells in good working order.

According to Nuala Byrne, a professor and health researcher at Tasmania University, the intermittent fasting strategy may weaken the starvation reaction and some of the body's adaptive thermogenesis processes, which means your body will cease fighting so hard to defend its fat stores.[19] This is encouraging news because adaptive thermogenesis makes it difficult for many of us to lose weight even with a rigorous diet and exercise regimen.

Intermittent fasting is an effective way of lowering your set point weight, losing excess fat and maintaining it, because it directly targets how your body produces and utilizes insulin. Since the discovery of insulin in 1921, its role in human metabolism continues to baffle scientists. Insulin plays a vital role in modulating fat metabolism. Insulin regulates fat uptake, fat storage, fat generation and fat breakdown. Elevated insulin levels are associated with obesity and people who take insulin to manage diabetes may experience weight gain. Insulin resistance is characterized by insulin receptor desensitization which impairs glucose uptake by cells in response to insulin stimulation. Therefore, individuals facing insulin resistance develop type 2 diabetes and many other diseases associated with it.

Insulin metabolism varies between individuals, which is another reason why some people are much more likely to become overweight and develop metabolic problems than someone living a similar lifestyle who metabolizes insulin effectively. After a substantial meal, it takes 4–6 hours for insulin levels to return to the baseline in an average non-diabetic person, implying that it takes 4–6 hours for the body to begin dipping into its fat stores for energy. If we constantly snack between meals, even if it's nuts or fruits, we're not allowing our insulin levels to return to that crucial baseline.

Though effective, intermittent fasting isn't the only way to improve our insulin metabolism, which will ultimately help reset your set point.

- Physical exercise improves insulin sensitivity and its effects are almost immediate.
- Quitting tobacco smoking may be a powerful step as tobacco causes insulin resistance.[20]
- Our stress hormone, cortisol, has a solid link to insulin resistance. Too much cortisol can impact our thyroid function, strongly influencing metabolism. Reducing stress and the amount of cortisol in our body can help to improve insulin sensitivity.
- Certain supplements may help to improve insulin sensitivity, such as berberine, magnesium and omega-3 fatty acids.
- Reducing ultra-processed and highly refined sugars in our diet will significantly reduce insulin resistance.
- Eating a diet high in whole and unprocessed foods, including nuts and fatty fish, improves insulin sensitivity.
- Getting enough good-quality sleep plays a significant role in insulin sensitivity.
- Reduced alcohol consumption and a regular bedtime routine, including a set bedtime, also helps.

Aside from improving insulin resistance, many health benefits have been associated with intermittent fasting. They include:

- Increased levels of human growth hormone (as much as fivefold). An increase in levels of this hormone facilitates fat burning and muscle gain.
- Controlled fasting triggers autophagy (cellular self-cleaning process).
- Increase in metabolic rate to anywhere between 3.6 per cent and 14 per cent.
- Reduction in belly fat.
- Protection against the development of type 2 diabetes.
- In diabetic patients, intermittent fasting can help prevent kidney damage (by reversing fatty kidney disease).
- Reduction of chronic low-grade inflammation.
- Improved blood pressure, total and LDL cholesterol, and blood triglycerides, all of which impact cardiac health.
- Increased levels of brain-derived neurotrophic factor (BDNF), a hormone whose deficiency has been linked to depression.
- Reduction in toxic side effects of chemotherapy and tumour growth in cancer patients.
- Increases both our lifespan and health span.

Despite some recent (2020 and 2022) studies published in the *New England Journal of Medicine* (NEJM) and *Journal of American Medical Association* (JAMA) showing that intermittent fasting did not necessarily lead to expected weight loss, we know that intermittent fasting works for many and we understand the mechanism by which it works.[21] The problem is that merely telling someone who has the habit of snacking multiple times a day to stop eating for several hours is impractical.[22] It is not easy for most to adopt a lifestyle that incorporates sixteen hours of fasting every day, let alone a more extreme version of prolonged fasting for over twenty-four hours.

People who have tried it and had good results still relapse to their prior unrestricted eating habits because their brains are wired to do so. Undiagnosed or untreated depression, stress and lack of sleep are barriers to long-term TRE success. In addition, social factors like spousal abuse, toxic relationships, burnout at work, deadlines and upcoming exams attract repeated exposure to highly palatable ultra-processed foods. These factors play into our ability to stick to a time-restricted eating pattern.

Our dependence on food extends beyond mere survival. Most of us depend on food for our emotional needs. When ultra-processed food (like any substance of abuse such as cocaine or nicotine) is ingested repeatedly, food dependence ensues. Once dependence sets in, discontinuing the substance (in this case, comfort food) results in withdrawal symptoms such as irritability, restlessness, tiredness and cravings. For instance, if you eat three to four times a day, your brain starts to depend on that particular schedule and quantity of food. Any attempt to cut down will result in food withdrawal symptoms.

Brain Rewiring

TRE rewires our brains by mitigating the brain's conditioned behaviour for withdrawal symptoms. Johns Hopkins neuroscientist Mark Mattson, PhD, has studied intermittent fasting for twenty-five years. His research shows that it can take two to four weeks before the body becomes accustomed to intermittent fasting.[23] He observed that research subjects who make it through the adjustment period tend to stick to the plan because they feel better and experience health benefits.

The cycle of food dependence that a person's brain has become accustomed to for many years or decades can be broken by those who challenge themselves by fasting a few times, usually for longer than eighteen hours. To succeed at TRE, you must identify the triggers that cause you to relapse into unhealthy eating habits. In addition, you may have to alter your feeding pattern to suit your life circumstances and health requirements, such as during an acute sickness.

Watch What You Eat during the Feeding Window

Snacking between meals is the hallmark of the modern lifestyle.[24] Even if you have the discipline not to eat during the set hours in a day, it's hard not to splurge and overindulge after the fasting period. During those precious feeding hours, one may indulge in comfort foods that are ultra-processed and unhealthy, rewarding oneself for enduring the fasting phase. After a few hours of fasting and depriving yourself of food, your brain's hunger centre goes into overdrive. It involves the right education, proper planning and expert supervision to eat healthy, nutritious meals during the feeding window.

Many assume that willpower and discipline are the answers to sticking to a strict diet regimen. This is not always true. Later in the book, we shall see how our willpower can easily be hijacked by savvy marketing and targeted advertisements from ultra-refined and fast-food companies.

* * *

Developing a Healthier Microbiome

Two options are available to 'cultivate' a favourable gut microbiome for maintaining a healthy weight. The first option is to take supplements or pills containing the good bacteria and hope that they'll integrate into your gut and befriend the good bacteria or evict the bad bacteria altogether, and make your gut their new home. The second option is to switch from an obesogenic diet to one high in wholefoods that naturally and favourably tilt the balance. Science is still evolving, but more evidence proves that the second approach is healthier and more sustainable.

Counteracting your body's innate tendency to defend its weight involves a multi-pronged approach, where you adopt a lifestyle that incorporates multiple techniques: intermittent fasting, the 10 per cent solution, cultivating a healthy microbiome and reducing ultra-processed foods are among the most important. Unfortunately, it is easier said than done, as changing your lifestyle to foster a healthy metabolism is against all the forces society has created.

Theoretically, we know how to manage our weight, but thanks to the abundance of ready-made, highly processed cheap foods and the desk-bound work life we have, maintaining a healthy weight is practically difficult for many, regardless of our chosen approach. We live in an obesogenic environment where sodas, pastries, chips and fried meals dominate the streets, malls and schools. Change only comes with an awareness of our conditioning.

How do we cultivate a healthy microbiome? We start by eliminating the bad and adding the good to our gut. We can attain a healthy microbiome by:

- Cutting down highly processed and packaged foods
- Eliminating artificial sweeteners
- Using antibiotics judiciously
- Limiting acid reflux medications to a short-term use
- Increasing wholefood, organic, plant-based food with high fibre content

Recognize and Reduce Adiposogens (Adiposity Generators)

Of the 80,000+ chemicals that have been registered for use in the US, some are toxic to animals and humans, while others disrupt the hormonal functioning of the body. These endocrine-disrupting chemicals have been linked to various diseases and some are involved in abnormal weight gain. They are referred to as obesogens. I call them adiposogens, the adiposity generators. The term obesogens was coined around 2006, based on the discovery that early developmental exposure to specific chemicals disrupted normal metabolic processes and elevated the risk of weight gain throughout life. They alter our gut microbiome and cause an imbalance of good and bad bacteria. They are everywhere, mostly in the routine household items that we use and the polluted air we breathe. Examples of these endocrine disruptors include:

1. Cigarette smoke
2. Air pollution
3. Tributyltin, a chemical commonly used as a fungicide and heat stabilizer in polyvinyl chloride (PVC) piping
4. Phthalates, chemicals used to soften many consumer products
5. Bisphenol A (BPA) used in making plastics and resins
6. Polychlorinated biphenyls (PCBs), industrial chemicals widely used in paints, cement, fluorescent light ballasts, sealants and adhesives
7. BPA linings on the inside of cans

Endocrine disruptors are thought to work in a variety of ways. They may alter the development of a person's fat cells by increasing fat storage capacity or the number of fat cells and changing the body's set point weight. These chemicals may also make it more challenging to maintain a healthy weight by altering how the body regulates feelings of hunger and fullness or amplifying the effects of high-fat and high-sugar diets.

How to Reduce Endocrine Disruptors?

Water

Use a filtration system that reduces exposure to chlorine. Limit (or eliminate) the use of plastic water bottles. Use a stainless steel or glass water bottle instead.

Food

Whenever possible, eat organic vegetables, meat and fruits. Many herbicides and pesticides contain these disruptors. The Environmental Working Group has lists of the dirty dozen and the clean fifteen.[25]

Use organic dairy products.[26]

Linings on cans contain BPA; therefore, avoid canned foods.[27]

Cooking utensils

Replace non-stick cookware with stainless steel or cast iron. Chemicals called perfluoroalkyl substances (PFAs) present in high concentrations in non-stick cookware was found to have endocrine-disrupting properties. They hinder the normal functioning of weight-regulating hormones such as insulin, oestrogen and thyroid. Studies have shown that people with higher PFA concentration in their blood had higher weight regain.[28]

Personal care and cosmetics

Perfumes, deodorants and other cosmetics products can expose you to endocrine disruptors such as parabens, phthalates, synthetic musks and many other potentially carcinogenic products, hence limit their use.

* * *

In summary, we know, in theory, how to manage our weight, but with an overabundance of ready-made, highly processed, cheap food combined with the relatively sedentary lifestyles most of us have, it is nearly impossible for many of us to defend a healthy weight, no matter what method we adopt. We all live in an obesogenic environment where our buildings have hidden staircases but instantly greet us with elevators and escalators.

We often point fingers at the individual for failing to lose weight and keep it off and fail to recognize that the problem is beyond just the individual. We have created an adiposity-generating environment, a self-sustaining catalyst for gaining unhealthy weight, which is almost impossible to reverse unless we recognize the root cause of the problem and take necessary actions.

At a Glance

➢ About 90 per cent of people who have lost a considerable amount of weight, regardless of the method used to do so, will gain most of it back in 1-5 years.
➢ Our bodies are genetically, hormonally and evolutionarily designed to defend weight. This ability was crucial to the survival of our species.
➢ The obesogenic environment we live in makes it extremely hard for an individual to maintain weight loss, despite their best efforts.

> ➢ By changing the environment we live in, we
>   have a better chance of maintaining our weight
>   loss, but this is a collective effort. Blaming
>   individuals for their failure is sheer injustice that
>   causes moral injury to the victim.

4

Weight-Loss Surgery—Far from an 'Easy Fix'

People with significant adiposity are at risk of serious complications such as uncontrolled blood pressure, high blood sugar or impending organ dysfunction such as heart, lung or kidney failure. Weight loss must occur fast in these emergency scenarios to reverse the consequences of metabolic illnesses and halt the development of more severe problems like a heart attack or stroke.

For individuals who have diligently tried to lose weight through nutrition, exercise and lifestyle changes without success, weight-loss surgery offers hope. However, this path is far from easy. Their bodies may struggle to adapt to the rapid weight loss post-surgery, and some weight may be regained afterwards. Many have felt fatigued and faced challenges during this demanding journey. Interestingly, most of them experienced additional frustration when their hopes were realized, as emotional battles arose in achieving their goals—a challenge often more significant than carrying excess weight. Some found that weight loss wasn't a cure-all as anticipated, and the stigma attached to weight-loss surgery still led to negative emotions.

* * *

Sophie walked into the clinic's waiting room accompanied by her mother. Her stomach began to rumble and her face reddened as she checked in at the reception desk. She had been on a liquid diet for two weeks and had eaten nothing except a few sparse sips of water since 10 p.m. the previous night. Her stomach grumbled again. She thought she saw the receptionist give her a sympathetic look but couldn't tell. Her mother took her hand in hers and squeezed it.

They settled in to wait—Sophie's cheeks turned red as she tried to fit herself into the armchair, feeling discomfort from its narrow arms against her hips. After a short while, her mother reached for a couple of magazines on the accent table and handed one to her. She accepted it, flipping through pages filled with celebrity news and advertisements featuring slender, radiant women, which only heightened her unease. The images in the magazines highlighted everything she felt she lacked—slim legs, defined cheekbones and much more. Setting the magazine aside, she switched to browsing social media on her phone. Her feed was filled with 'before and after' photos of people who had undergone weight-loss surgery. 'Soon, I'll have my own "after" picture,' she whispered to herself.

Sophie was facing the scariest challenge of her life. She was about to have a section of her tummy chopped off and sewn into a smaller sack.

Sophie used to play soccer regularly ever since she was a kid. In her final year of college, she discontinued soccer to focus on her exams, only to observe an ever-increasing weight in the years that followed. The peak of her weight gain occurred when her boyfriend of six years broke up with her after they graduated from college. They had been best friends since elementary school and did everything together. Even after graduating from high school and enrolling in different colleges, they tirelessly communicated every night and spent every weekend together. In addition, they had planned on taking a year off after graduation to travel. Unfortunately, they broke up before then and he went on the planned trip alone. Following the sudden change of events, Sophie moved back in with her parents. She was lonely and suffered from depression. This was when she found comfort in junk food and indulged in it uncontrollably, causing her to gain weight rapidly.

Fast forward to a few years later, when she was twenty-seven years old. Standing at 5'4" and weighing 120 kg, Sophie was considered morbidly obese; she had type 2 diabetes, high blood pressure, PCOS, sleep apnea, joint pains and infertility at such a young age. Her medical providers recommended that she diet and exercise, but nothing worked despite her best efforts to follow the diet and exercise regime. The comorbidities that accompanied her adiposity made her unfit to work for over a year.

Sophie's primary care physician initially 'managed' her illnesses by prescribing drugs. She and her doctor agreed that her metabolic health was more important than her weight. If left untreated, it would result in organ failures including the heart, kidney, liver and others, eventually leading to incapacitation or premature death. Given that the only thing that could save her was surgery, her primary-care physician referred her to a bariatric surgeon in the hopes of reversing her illnesses due to obesity. Sophie is one of the quarter-million people in the United States who get weight-loss surgery every year.

She mumbled incoherently and choked on her sobs as she sat in the waiting room. This surgery was her best shot and the only thread of hope she held on to—while she was nervous and scared, she was excited to feel normal again, and see improvements in her health and overall quality of life. She had already read everything her doctor recommended. Nevertheless, the surgery she was about to undergo was irreversible and she could never know fully how it would change her life.

Disease Management

The term patient conjures up a vision of passive suffering. It is derived from the Latin *patiens*, from *patior*, meaning to suffer or bear.[1] Today's medical-industrial complex turns *people* into *patients* who are hooked to lifelong medications.

Medical students in the late 1990s were taught that type 2 diabetes and hypertension are irreversible diseases. You can only manage them by using drugs and 'eating less, exercising more'. Medical doctors were trained to use drugs to 'maintain' such chronic illnesses, while the job of a nutritionist was to advise patients on diet and nutrition. Making lifestyle alterations to treat chronic illnesses played second fiddle to drug therapy. It was difficult to ask people to change their behaviour but writing a prescription was easy. It was also too time-consuming and laborious for busy doctors to coach patients on making lifestyle adjustments to address a medical condition.

For a long time, neither research studies nor medical practices considered the idea of 'reversing' a chronic disease such as diabetes or high blood pressure. In the early 1950s, a positive change occurred in the practice of medicine as physicians began identifying measures to prevent an illness from occurring in the first place, alongside treating the symptoms of an illness once it arose. The notion of disease prevention in modern Western medicine originally stemmed from a study of infectious diseases but was later applied to other non-communicable diseases. Dr E. Gurney Clark, an epidemiologist at Columbia University in New York, wrote a groundbreaking article in 1954 entitled 'Natural History of Syphilis and Levels of Prevention', describing syphilis from a preventive standpoint.[2] Just a year before the publication of this article, Clark had co-authored the *Textbook of Preventive Medicine* with Dr Hugh R. Leavell of Harvard, which is still used as a valuable resource today.[3]

The impact of Leavell and Clark's work was so significant that the concept of preventing and then managing diseases became the standard. However, doctors have never focused on reversing chronic diseases.

Disease Reversal

In 1992, Dr Walter Pories, a bariatric surgeon, wrote his landmark paper, 'Is Type II Diabetes Mellitus (NIDDM) a Surgical Disease?'.[4] That marked the foundation for the idea that surgery could treat non-surgical diseases.

Traditionally, the main aim of surgery was centred around anatomy. Its purpose was to eliminate a tumour, address a cataract, remove an infected organ like the appendix or gall bladder, halt bleeding from a ruptured aneurysm, perform amputations for infected limb parts and similar procedures. Pories' research served as a watershed moment in the entire field of medicine as it was the first time a surgery was used primarily to enhance the body's metabolism.

In 1995, Pories published another article, alongside his research team, entitled, 'Who Would Have Thought It? An Operation Proves to Be the Most Effective Therapy for Adult-Onset Diabetes Mellitus', that proved to be a major milestone.[5] Since then, much evidence has supported that bariatric surgery has the potential to improve several metabolic diseases and even *cure* them, so much so that weight-loss surgery is increasingly known as metabolic surgery.

Surgeons were ecstatic, not just because they had created a novel surgical procedure, but because it instilled a sense of great pride in them. From antiquity until medieval times, surgeons were placed on a lower rung than clergy physicians, who considered the practice of surgery beneath their dignity. Barber surgeons were in charge of procedures like bloodletting, amputation and tooth extraction. During medieval times, surgeons were called 'barbers' because they performed surgical procedures along with tasks like hair-cutting, shaving and administering enemas, which were considered less dignified for medical practitioners. The division between surgeons and physicians persisted until surgeons proved their ability to address issues that physicians couldn't, and to do so more efficiently.

The American Society for Bariatric Surgery (ASBS) was founded in 1983.[6] In 2009, it was renamed the American Society for Metabolic and Bariatric Surgery (ASMBS) because many were convinced that surgeons, not physicians, could steer the fate of medicine in curing many chronic diseases, which was witnessed by millions in the national media and on the international stage.

Metabolic Surgery

Several different bariatric procedures have been developed in recent years. Still, they all share the same principle—reducing the absorption of food through the gastrointestinal (GI) tract, either by restricting the amount of food consumed or by decreasing the amount of digested food absorbed into circulation. Currently, the two most effective procedures in this regard are Roux-en-Y gastric bypass (RYGB) and vertical sleeve gastrectomy (VSG).

1. Roux-en-Y gastric bypass (RYGB)

In RYGB, the gastrointestinal tract is altered such that swallowed food exits the oesophagus and enters the small intestine directly, bypassing the stomach altogether.

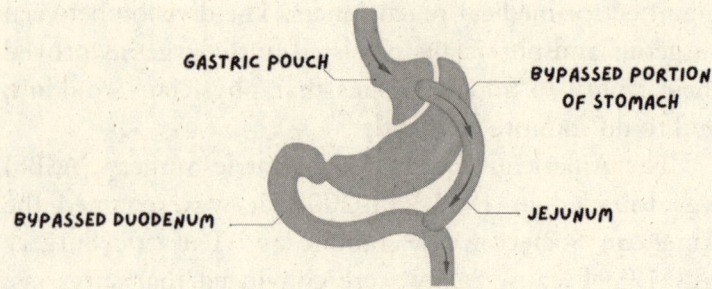

Figure 4.1: Gastric Bypass

2. Vertical sleeve gastrectomy (VSG)

In VSG, most of the stomach is surgically removed. Only a thin cylinder of stomach tissue remains between the oesophagus and the start of the intestines. Thus, food in RYGBs the stomach and the first half of the small intestine completely, but food in VSG passes via a smaller stomach and travels the entire length of the intestine.

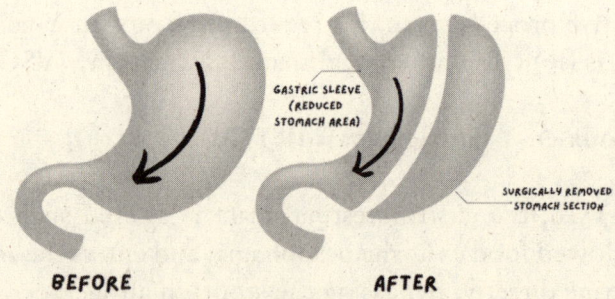

Figure 4.2: Vertical sleeve Gastrectomy

Both result in a reduction in food intake and absorption. The long-term weight loss and improvements in metabolic and health indices lead to longer lives and, most importantly, an improved quality of life.

While it was initially thought that the weight loss experienced after the surgery was either due to reduced absorption of food because of restricted stomach size or changes in satiety hormones, neither theory has been proven. Laboratories worldwide are trying to answer the question: How does bariatric surgery work? Do RYGB or VSG procedures somehow trick the weight-regulatory process in the brain? We know the surgery works but are still unsure as to how it works.

What is particularly striking is that despite the different ways of rerouting swallowed food, both procedures result in comparable improvements in body weight, diabetes and other metabolic symptoms. Body fat, in particular, settles at a new and considerably lower weight, as if the body fat's set point thermostat was lowered.

Bariatric surgery was an eureka moment for doctors regarding the digestive system and human metabolism, with surgical treatment of metabolic disorders being a game changer in the medical field.[7]

Before Pories' publications, even the medical community mocked the idea of disease reversal. It was weight loss through a surgical intervention that opened up new vistas in the field of medicine, not just in the treatment of obesity. Individuals who have undergone weight-loss surgery and lost tremendous weight have been able to reverse many illnesses such as diabetes, high blood pressure, high lipids, sleep apnea,

PCOS, fatty liver, asthma, male hypogonadism, female infertility, urinary incontinence, acid reflux, depression, osteoarthritis and more.[8]

Several patients who have undergone gastric bypass surgery have spoken publicly about the genuine post-surgery reversal of the disease.

'I weighed almost 350 pounds [159 kg] before [gastric bypass] surgery,' Kevin Brown said. 'I have type 2 diabetes and was on the verge of needing insulin shots. I was on two different types of diabetes meds and a blood pressure medication. I haven't had any prescriptions since my operation.'[9]

'Bypass surgery was the best thing I ever did!' exclaimed Natalia Laforce. 'I had significant arthritis in my neck, back, and feet and severe sleep apnea. I had reached a point where I was unable to walk. I was able to jog after my surgery. I ascended a peak. I occasionally experience discomfort, but it's nothing like it was.' She continued, 'My legs aren't as bloated as they used to be. My thyroid has stabilized. My blood sugars are normal. My blood pressure is within normal limits. My cholesterol level is good.'[10]

Bariatric Surgery—Not an Infallible Cure

Bariatric surgery is, however, not a cure-all procedure—many people continue to struggle even after going under the knife. In recent years, published research has demonstrated that it is difficult for bariatric surgery patients to sustain their weight loss, even if they had initially succeeded. In a meta-analysis of twenty-nine long-term weight-loss studies, more than 50 per cent of the lost weight was regained within two years, and more than 80 per cent of lost weight was regained by five years. Moreover, about 20 per cent of bariatric surgery patients fail to lose at least 50 per cent of their excess body weight.

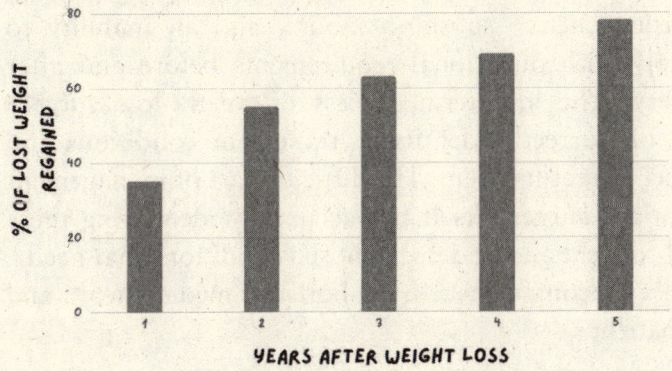

Figure 4.3: Percentage of Annual Weight Regain After Initial Loss

Why Do Most Weight-loss Surgeries Fail in the Long Term (after Ten Years)?

Many theories explain why this can happen. One of the theories stated that patients may begin to gradually increase their eating some time after the surgery, causing their stomachs to expand again. Although many patients cannot eat as much after the surgery, they continue to consume high numbers of excess calories in the form of sugary drinks, against the advice of their medical team. As a result, we now have novel surgeries that promise weight loss (of the regained weight) following bariatric surgery. For many, the struggle appears to be never-ending.

The success of any weight-loss surgery largely depends on the patient's lifestyle and psychological state *before* the surgery. Conditions where a weight-loss surgery will result in high failure rates are poorly controlled psychiatric illnesses (such as major depression), eating disorders, active substance abuse, and an inability to comply with nutritional requirements before and after surgery. The long-term success of weight-loss surgery rests on correctly identifying these four conditions and properly treating them. The difficult part of management is not the surgery itself but accurately identifying these hard-to-treat and under-diagnosed conditions that need a long-term commitment from both the medical team and the patient.

Surgery Aftermath: The Second Stigma

'Did you know that when an obese person undergoes bariatric surgery, it's extremely common to have body dysmorphia? Although I weigh 170 pounds [77 kg], I still see myself as 300 pounds [136 kg] in the mirror. (Yes, I'm in therapy for it.) So doing jumping jacks might have to wait for now,' shared one of my nurse friends who recently had weight-loss surgery.

Weight-loss surgery can change the lives of obese people for the better. However, it carries its own stigma. In a recent study, a group of people were shown images of lean men and women and asked to rate their impression of that individual on various characteristics.[11] They were then shown pictures of the same person before their weight loss. The participants rated individuals who lost weight through surgery as lazier, sloppier, less competent and sociable, less attractive, and following less healthy eating habits. By comparison, the individuals who lost weight through diet and exercise were not rated so harshly. Participants shared the opinion that individuals who lost weight due to surgery had 'cheated' and carried less responsibility for their weight loss than their counterparts who dieted and exercised.

While many people enjoy genuine improvements in their quality of life due to their surgery, numerous hardships still exist. If you rapidly lost a lot of weight primarily through weight-loss surgery, you are prone to encounter the following challenges:

1. Your mind hasn't adjusted to your new body.
2. When someone compliments you on your weight-loss accomplishments, you may not appreciate it or may even feel awful about it because it constantly reminds you of your shortcomings.
3. You have a distorted body image after losing considerable weight post-surgery. Almost everyone who undergoes weight-loss surgery encounters this problem. Fortunately, this gets better over time as the overweight version fades from your consciousness and your brain adjusts to the new thinner version.

'I tell patients before their operation to think about this: You have this weight problem that is not only physical but also psychological and emotional,' says Neely Williams, who had bariatric surgery. She further adds, 'You've been labelled and now that you've had this surgery, extraordinary things begin to happen: you lose weight and appear to be in fantastic shape. Eighteen months, twenty-four months pass and if you haven't been able to find new ways of living your life, you're back to doing what you were doing before the operation and the weight returns. If that happens, you'll have a double problem: you gained weight, lost it and now you've gained it back—you'll be stigmatized twice.'[12]

Another bariatric surgery patient, Chloe Greenlee, says, 'Society stigmatizes everything about obesity.' She further explains, 'They encourage people to lose weight, but nobody is pleased when we undergo surgery. I was the same way at first: I felt embarrassed to be having surgery. It may be the easy way out, but it is not.[13] It entailed a significant adjustment in my eating and exercising habits.'[14]

Unfortunately, obesity and weight loss seem to be a no-win situation for many people. The public's impression of weight-loss surgery reflects their perception of obesity's willpower weakness. According to Dr Eric DeMaria, president of the ASMBS, 'You're essentially admitting to being a personal failure as a human being because you can't reduce weight on your own.'[15]

Far From an 'Easy Fix'

Weight-loss surgery is not a magical cure-all and neither is it the 'easy fix'. Instead, it is better to consider it as a piece of the puzzle towards achieving a healthy weight and reducing the risk of obesity-related comorbid complications. The procedure itself carries risks. In fact, the post-surgery recovery period is rather long, and patients can expect to experience pain and discomfort throughout their post-op recovery. In addition, everyone who undergoes surgery *still has to diet*. Patients are restricted to a liquid-only diet for the first two weeks after surgery, followed by soft foods as they build up to reintroduce solid foods into their regime.

Following surgery, patients are urged to practise the following:[16]

- Eat smaller portions of meals very slowly. Each meal should take at least thirty minutes.
- Drink plenty of water before and after meals, but not within thirty minutes after eating, as this can trigger 'dumping syndrome', a set of symptoms that includes diarrhea, nausea and feeling light-headed or exhausted due to food flowing too quickly from the stomach to the duodenum.
- Take small bites and chew thoroughly to avoid blockages of the small intestine.
- Avoid foods that are high in fats and sugar as they can contribute to dumping syndrome. That means no chips, cakes, candy, sodas or chocolate, and most foods rich in carbohydrates, such as bread, pasta, rice and potatoes. Instead, opt for a high-protein diet.

The decision to undergo surgery is one with life-changing consequences. Transformation is for the better, but it does not occur without sacrifice, hard work and the patient's commitment to their health. It could be the boost people need to get a leg-up on their journey to a healthy weight, manage illnesses like type 2 diabetes, lower their risk of developing diseases like heart disease, extend their lifespan, as well as improve their quality of life, boost their self-esteem, and discover new pathways for growth.

Weight-loss surgery is not a 'cheat' card for losing weight. One out of every ten weight-loss surgery patients will regain the weight they lost, and surgeons cannot determine who will succeed and who will fail to meet their post-surgical goals. Some people find that the surgery has significantly reduced their hunger and desire. In contrast, others find it difficult to lose weight even after a section of their stomach has been removed.

Weight-loss surgery should be considered a last resort, only after all other weight-loss methods have been attempted and failed. However, maintaining the strict post-surgery regimen is also a challenging task. The surgery can serve as motivation to adhere to a rigorous daily diet routine, but sustaining this discipline for several years requires both personal determination and a supportive lifestyle environment.

* * *

It has been three years since Sophie's surgery. Today, she weighs 155 pounds (70 kg), down from the initial 265 pounds (120 kg). Six months after her surgery, she returned to the job she loved as a teacher, and within a year, she was back to playing soccer. After eighteen months post-op, she no longer had to take medication for her type 2 diabetes. She regularly goes to her physician for check-ups, and the good news is that her diabetes seems to be reversed. Furthermore, her ovaries began functioning normally again thanks to the weight loss, significantly improving her fertility. She and her fiancé, Stephen, expect their first baby in the new year.

Sophie's journey wasn't linear. At one point, she gained back 27 kg and was forced to take some time off work due to its toll on her mental health. With her waning motivation and it being infinitely easier to grab something from the freezer aisle than to prepare fresh food, Sophie slipped back into her old habits. Whenever her mood was low and her self-esteem was on the floor, she grabbed takeout and took a mental break from her strict diet and exercise programme. During a low period, she was unmotivated to go to the gym or join her soccer team on the pitch. It was more accessible to snack on pre-packaged foods than to prepare snacks in the mornings. It took speaking to a therapist and completing twelve weeks of cognitive-behavioural therapy (CBT) to help get her back on track again, and to the place she is today.

* * *

Losing Weight Doesn't Always Lessen the Load We Carry

Aside from the emotional baggage left after significant weight loss, some people are left with a physical reminder of the weight they once carried. Shedding excess weight leaves a lasting impression on the body—stretch marks and loose skin become a constant reminder of shame on an outstanding achievement. People may even intentionally decide to regain some weight to feel 'full' and 'complete' again.

Some people have reported feeling uneasy when flirted with since they aren't used to well-intentioned flirting and suspect they are being mocked. Psychologist Janis Rosenberg, PhD, recalls that one of her clients perceived positive attention from men as 'an assault'.[17] Entitled comments from purportedly well-meaning passers-by only aggravated her further. Most people tend to feel uncomfortable with this increased attention. Over time, these comments lay a steady, unrelenting assault on the psyche of a person who is getting used to his/her new weight.

Another practical challenge for many people after losing weight is the need to shop for new clothes to fit their new frames. Having spent years buying plus-sized clothing or simply choosing the largest size available to accommodate their shape, the thought of having to go shopping can be extremely challenging and off-putting for many. Even seeing yourself strip down in a dressing room mirror may bring up feelings of dread. Getting a new bra fitting can be particularly intimidating for women. Therefore, people may spend months wearing their old, oversized clothing as they get used to their new bodies.

'When I visit stalls and try on clothes, I cry by myself in the changing room,' a young woman wrote on the popular community site Reddit. 'I don't like what I see; my arms, stomach, boobs, legs; clothes never fit me well. I turn away from the mirror so I don't have to look in it since all I can think of is how ugly I am.'[18] Another woman commented on the same forum, 'I'm in serious need of new clothes. Because of my recent weight loss, very little of what I possess fits me well, and the majority of what I own are two-year-old tank tops. Every time I go to the mall to buy something, I look in the mirrors and think of how terrible I appear.'

Weight loss is a physiological process, but it is more than simply lowering calorie intake and upping energy output. Do it too fast and the body will quickly revert to a famine response, making it nearly impossible to keep the weight off. It has been demonstrated that those who experience the yo-yo effect over periods of dieting are less likely to successfully maintain their weight loss in the long run.

No Standard Road Map for Weight Loss

Losing weight is a journey but it is not as simple as choosing your mode of transport and following the signposts. Nobody can guarantee that you will successfully get to 68 kg from 127 kg. Even if a diet is rigorously outlined with a clear timeline and step-by-step instructions, our bodies are different. Given how unpredictable the human body is, a diet that works for one person is not guaranteed to work for another. Some people may be physiologically predestined to fail in their efforts, no matter how many different diets they try. Those who do reach their goals will likely not have arrived unscathed.

When it comes to losing weight, we have various tools and methods available, and it's important for individuals and medical professionals to work closely together to determine the best approach, being open to adjusting the plan if challenges arise. Above all, patients should prioritize their physical, mental and emotional well-being throughout their weight-loss journey. Just as lifestyle changes are crucial for maintaining weight loss, support for mental health is equally essential after shedding weight.

This is a learning curve for patients and medical professionals alike. We need to rewrite the playbook of how we approach dieting and weight loss, and reconsider our expectations regarding each person's individuality and needs. We must also recognize that some people will get lost a few times en route to their destination.

As a society, we are very quick to judge. We see a perceived problem and the first thing we do is assign blame. People suffering from obesity wear their malady plainly for all to see and bear the brunt of the stigma associated with that daily. They had to overcome numerous obstacles, such as admitting they had a problem and seeking counselling, attempting to reduce weight on their own through diet and exercise, failing and suffering the mental toll, and finally making the difficult decision to undergo surgery.

As individuals persist in their valiant struggle, carving paths of transformation through profound personal changes and unwavering sacrifices to shed weight, the journey doesn't cease at the pinnacle of accomplishment. They encounter a world quick to pass judgment, a society that often casts its critical gaze without comprehending the internal battles waged. Amid our pursuit to combat obesity, a resounding imperative emerges—one that impels us to delve deeper into the heart of the matter, to scrutinize the very fabric of society that weaves this intricate tapestry of challenges.

At a Glance

❖ Sustained weight loss can be difficult for some bariatric surgery patients, even if they initially succeed.

❖ The stigma surrounding the surgery is a barrier to recovery, just as the stigma towards obesity is a barrier to people seeking help in the first place.

❖ Losing weight is the first challenge. Accepting your new body is the second and potentially greater mountain to climb.

5

Are We Food Addicts?

I once had the opportunity to care for Joe, a man in his late forties, who was admitted to the hospital for the treatment of pneumonia. Unfortunately, his recovery turned out to be more challenging and prolonged than expected. His excessive weight led to respiratory challenges, a complication termed obesity hypoventilation syndrome. As he improved and prepared to leave the hospital, I knew I couldn't ignore the topic of his weight. At 5′9″, he carried a weight of 127 kg. Starting the conversation, I braced myself for any discomfort, but to my surprise, Joe welcomed the discussion. It was like addressing 'the elephant in the room', and he appreciated that I cared enough to have an open and supportive conversation about it.

'Doc, I know I am obese, but it's not like I want to be,' he started. 'I'll be honest. Once I start eating, I can't stop. I could try to eat healthier, but the moment I crave something, I must eat it. I feel like a prisoner; I constantly eat fries, drink a lot of soda, and if I start on a pizza, all hell breaks loose. Every day I wake, the first thing that pops into my mind is food. I feel a rush when I start eating and I literally can't stop till my stomach is about to burst. Guilt and shame engulf me after this, but I still do it again. The only time I don't eat is when I'm asleep. Every once in a while, I muster my willpower and control my eating, but the old habits resurface after a day. I want to change. I don't want to be back here again in a few months; I want to stop this cycle and get healthy, but I don't think it's possible.'

Compare him to another patient I treated a few days earlier, Shawn, who was battling heroin addiction. Shawn narrated how he woke up every morning thinking about heroin to the extent that it interfered with his daily life. He tried multiple times to quit but with no success. He further explained how he lost his job due to his addiction. Despite all this, he still couldn't stop using it. Shawn felt hopeless.

Joe and Shawn were both stuck in a cycle they cannot break. Both were addicted to a substance, heroin and food, which negatively impacted their lives in a plethora of ways.

* * *

Food processing has played a pivotal role in enabling our species to flourish, influencing the development of numerous civilizations. Moreover, cooking remains a central delight for humans, forming the bedrock of cultures through delectable dishes, festive gatherings, indulgent treats and grand banquets. Anthropologists regard cooking and cuisine as vital cultural markers within societies. Bonds of friendship and matrimony have often been sealed over shared meals, fine wines and beverages.

Our lives are intimately associated with food. Sometimes, we eat to regulate our mood. In turn, our mood can also control our food habits. Some of us lose our appetites in the face of stress, while others overeat in response to stressful situations. Life events, break-ups, conflicts, loneliness or tasks like deadlines or school exams can compel us to consume mood-enhancing, carbohydrate-rich foods and drinks to alleviate distress, fill the emotional void and provide comfort. We can feel the sense of wholesomeness and the feeling of satiation as quickly as two minutes after the first bite of these comfort foods such as candy bars, soda, cookies and other savoury snacks. The addictive nature of such foods, coupled with the satisfaction we feel upon eating them, causes us to continue eating far beyond our satiation level. Any mood-altering experience has the capacity to influence our eating patterns. For instance, a study revealed that participants ate more chocolate after viewing a distressing film than an emotionally neutral film.[1]

Eating comfort food with family is a joy and a reason to celebrate. Are you saying I should let go of the experience?

Indeed, food serves as a comforting refuge during times of stress, yet it's equally common for us to turn to it in moments of success. Whether to soothe our lows or to reward our highs, food holds a special place as a balm for our emotions.

The neurological underpinnings behind an intense longing for palatable food intrigued a few psychologists and neuroscientists, especially since the 1980s. Canadian scientist Harvey Weingarten conducted an experiment where he rang a bell while feeding his lab rats and observed that the rats began to associate the sound of the ringing bell with food—much like Pavlov's dogs.[2] But when Weingarten gave the rats a meal when they weren't hungry, they ignored the food completely despite seeing it, until he rang the bell. Weingarten discovered that the rats gobbled up the food despite showing no initial interest in dining. He published his observations in *Science* in 1983. Subsequent researchers have extrapolated Weingarten's findings to human behaviour. 'The experiment demonstrates how cues in our environment influence what we eat and how much,' observed Dana Small, a brain researcher and psychologist who heads the Modern Diet and Physiology Research lab at Yale University's School of Medicine.[3] According to Professor Small, the results of the experiment proved that an individual can overeat beyond the sense of satiety because of his uncontrollable urge to eat even though he is no longer hungry.

Hara Hachi Bu

Hara Hachi Bu, a Japanese phrase, translates to consuming food until you feel 80 per cent full, leaving your stomach only eight parts occupied.[4] This practice is prevalent in Okinawa, where residents strive to adhere to this principle. Okinawans boast one of the world's longest life expectancies and enjoy notably low rates of heart disease, cancers, stroke and obesity. Numerous epidemiological studies on this community have led health experts to recommend the 80 per cent rule to Westerners.

But how can we achieve the 80 per cent fullness? The process involves estimating the amount of food that would make us entirely full and then consuming only 80 per cent of that portion. The crucial aspect is to eat slowly and attentively. The rationale is that eating at a leisurely pace allows your mind to register the amount consumed. It typically takes around twenty minutes for your brain to catch up with your stomach's content, so the aim is to spend that time eating the 80 per cent portion that satisfies your hunger.

According to the traditional Indian medicine, Ayurveda, one *anjali* (two handfuls) of food is the recommended quantity to eat for the main meal. A person's stomach is estimated to have three anjali capacities, which means one anjali can be used for food, the other for water, and the third for air to facilitate the churning of the food and water. The rationale behind this instruction is that people frequently leave little or no space in their stomachs for air or even water, overburdening the digestive process. When we eat until we are almost

100 per cent full, our stomach expands due to the stretch reflex, resulting in a sensation of contentment. On the other hand, as the size of the stomach increases, the urge for food increases consequently and the vicious cycle continues.

Ayurveda recommends keeping your stomach less packed to gain maximum satisfaction from life. Never eat until you're completely satisfied.

The Japanese and Indians got it right. However, when we try to put these valuable instructions into practice, we find it challenging to follow them. Many people who suffer from obesity also suffer from faulty satiety signalling in their brains. Worst of all, this flawed satiety mechanism is rarely under our conscious control. It is influenced and amplified by factors beyond our own will.

The problem lies in how our body processes naturally occurring food items. Our gut spends more time and energy extracting nutrients from fruits and vegetables in their natural or minimally processed form than highly processed and refined foods. This absorption rate is largely dependent on our degree of satiety.

Satiation and Satiety

Satiation means satisfying our hunger and ending the desire to continue eating once we are full. Satiety is a physical feeling of fullness experienced after eating that prevents one from eating any more before hunger returns. Both are necessary to determine how much we consume and when to stop consuming.

Satiety is a seemingly simple phenomenon but requires a complex symphony of neurohormonal orchestration. It has to occur at an appropriate time with the appropriate amount of food in the stomach to achieve an optimum level of nutrition—not too much, not too little. Impaired satiety leads to overconsumption of food beyond our homeostatic needs.

The foods we choose and the amounts we consume play a pivotal role in determining our sense of fullness. When we consume carbohydrates and our stomach stretches, an intricate dance of hormones comes into play. These hormones, including cholecystokinin, glucagon-like peptide 1, oxyntomodulin and peptide YY, work as appetite regulators, signalling us to either slow down or halt our eating.[5] They originate predominantly in a section of our small intestine called the ileum. As our stomach expands and reaches satiety, our intestines send a message to our brain, indicating that it's time to stop eating. This phenomenon, known as intestinal satiety, begins with the first bite and concludes in the small intestine. However, the consumption of excessive comfort foods, which often contain predigested nutrients, can disrupt this intricate signalling mechanism.

Many individuals with obesity also experience disrupted satiety signals in their brain. Unfortunately, this impaired satiety response is often beyond our conscious influence.

When highly processed food is ingested, it is absorbed intensely in the earlier part of the gut and quickly assimilated into the blood. As a result, negligible amounts of nutrients reach the latter part of the small gut, where the intestinal satiety centres are predominantly located. Since a negligible amount of nutrients reach the intestinal satiety centre, it will release little to no satiety hormones to signal the brain to stop consuming. Owing to this disruption of gut–brain signalling, the person continues eating far beyond the point of the stomach being full. At this point, it is no longer hunger that motivates eating but gluttony.

Contrary to the idea that gluttony (originating from the Latin word *gluttire*, meaning 'to gulp down')[6] is a sinful behaviour, it actually serves as a protective mechanism. Our ancient hunter–gatherer bodies and brains developed this trait over millions of years of evolution to safeguard against potential food shortages, even though such scarcities are now unlikely. Our struggle to recognize when to cease eating arises because the foods we consume aren't inherently designed to signal when we're satisfied. This disconnection in our feeding signals can result in overeating, eventually contributing to the development of obesity.

As a society, we take emotional eating[7] very lightly. It is largely considered acceptable to manage our emotions by eating comfort food. Which one of us wasn't offered a lollipop at the doctor's office or a bowl of ice cream after a tough day at school? Which of us hasn't continued to comfort ourselves in this way into our adult lives? However, just as consuming recreational drugs often lead to drug dependency, palatable food-seeking often culminates in compulsive eating and, ultimately, a food addiction with negative health outcomes like obesity. The most interesting part of this is that our satiety can be easily hacked and it starts by seducing our taste buds.

> When gut–brain signalling is disrupted, the person might keep eating even after their stomach is full. At this stage, eating is driven not by hunger but by overindulgence.

Hacking Our Taste Mechanism

Of course, most of us want to consume foods that offer excellent nutritional value. However, who among us truly enjoys eating something devoid of flavour every day, no matter how nutritious it might be? Unfortunately, palatability is determined by the taste of the food, not its nutritional value. We don't enjoy food for what it does after it's digested and assimilated into our blood; we relish food for its taste and the experience of savouring it while it's in our mouths.

The human mouth contains approximately 5000 to 10,000 taste buds, and each taste bud is composed of 50–100 taste receptor cells. In total, there are around 2,50,000 to 1 million taste receptors that trigger sensations like sweet, salty, sour and bitter in response to the palatability of what we eat. Each taste has its specific receptor in the mouth.

Beyond taste, various receptors that sense temperature, consistency and texture of food evoke feelings of pleasure and comfort, enhancing the palatability of certain foods. Apart from the basic tastes, the richness or heartiness of food also impacts our emotional state before eating and can shape our meal experience. The setting also matters— our eating behaviour differs at a dining table versus in a car. Ultimately, our enjoyment of food is a multifaceted interplay between biology, culture, social influences, socio-economic status and the environment.

The dietary guidelines recommended by professional organizations have all advised us for the longest time to minimize eating comfort foods like cakes, cookies, chips or pizzas. Still, we all understand how challenging it is to eat just one cookie or a handful of chips, even when we've promised ourselves otherwise. Guilt soon sets in but you still can't help yourself the next time around, even when it is a short time later.

Appetite isn't a singular notion; it encompasses different appetites for various nutrients and tastes. Our appetite varies widely, spanning from refined carbohydrates to natural foods. Manufacturers of ultra-processed foods capitalize on our unfulfilled cravings.

Our response to controlling how much food we consume is deeply sophisticated. This seemingly simple process that we think is in our conscious control has an evolutionary mechanism. Taste is a phenomenon that has evolved to help us distinguish between safe and unsafe foods. Our brains go to great lengths not just for taste but also for survival. A sour taste in milk or meat, for instance, signals that the food is rotten and should be avoided. Spoiled food releases certain noxious chemicals detected by our taste receptors as unsavoury, thus preventing us from eating something that could cause us to feel unwell. Foods that provide immediate energy for humans are usually sweet, signalling an evolutionary taste preference for carbohydrates.

Our brain has evolved to safeguard the perpetuation of our species. However, this sophistication can be manipulated. The sweetness receptors on our tongues can be deceived by sweet-tasting substances like saccharin or aspartame, commonly known as artificial sweeteners. These substances replicate sweetness and activate the reward centres in our brains, elevating the appeal of otherwise ordinary foods when combined with them. While we recognize that processed wheat or flour lacks taste by itself, when paired with artificial sugars, it transforms into a delectable cookie.

Sugar isn't the only weapon in the arsenal. Food scientists can make a substance extremely flavourful by adding a combination of tastes like salty and sour, sweet and salty, sweet and savoury etc.[8] By enhancing the food compounds with just the right amount of taste combinations, a 'bliss point' can be achieved, where we can dupe the brain into believing it is receiving a new kind of reward, which is definitely more rewarding than a single taste.[9] By mixing and matching different threshold levels of substances, manipulating ingredients and tinkering with their chemistry, we can target products towards a whole population or specific subset (like children or adolescents), making them addicted to our product.

What's truly unsettling is that the higher our intake of refined sugar, the stronger our cravings become. Professor Anthony Sclafani, a nutritionist at New York University who investigates appetite and weight gain, made an intriguing discovery in his studies with lab rats.[10] When fed regular rat food, these rats barely gained weight. But, when they were given highly processed foods, they quickly gained excess weight. Additionally, their desire for sweet foods seemed insatiable, persisting even after they were already full.

The unfortunate truth is that your palate is never truly satisfied. When you indulge in something delicious, you experience a moment of delightful fulfilment, but it fades rapidly and the pattern repeats. Hunger re-emerges as swiftly as it disappears. Numerous individuals find themselves caught in this cycle, repeatedly giving in to cravings throughout the day.[11] Feelings of guilt arise for the perceived lack of self-control and promises to improve are made, yet the cycle persists. For many, food addiction is a reality, varying only in its intensity.

By skilfully blending food compounds with precise taste combinations, a culinary 'bliss point' can be achieved. This artful deception convinces the brain that it's experiencing a fresh and more gratifying reward, surpassing the allure of a solitary taste.

When Sugar Is More Rewarding than Cocaine

The rapid increase in obesity has prompted a keen interest in understanding the parallels between substance abuse disorders and excessive food consumption, including the impact of external cues and the formation of habits. Research now firmly establishes that addiction to highly processed foods, such as pizzas, cookies, chocolate and chips, carries a similar addictive potential as substances like cocaine. On the other hand, natural foods like fruits and vegetables show minimal addictive traits. Unlike our intense cravings for fried, salty and sugary foods, there's no comparable desire for fruits or vegetables.

Repeated eating of some highly palatable foods encourages habit-forming behaviours in humans, promoting hedonic hunger even more. Hedonic hunger is the desire to eat for pleasure, which means that people eat more than their homeostatic demands, making it another maladaptive food intake habit.[12]

When scientists exposed test animals to highly processed foods such as cheesecake and cookies, they exhibited neurobiological dysfunction in the dopamine system and behavioural changes such as binge eating, consistent with addiction. These studies exposed the 'dark' side of addiction, illustrating how subjects exposed to these highly processed foods showed negative mood states such as anhedonia, an inability to feel pleasure in normally pleasurable activities, and anxiety when their access to these foods was restricted. The study's participants repeatedly consumed these foods to reduce these negative emotional states and avoid a withdrawal-like state experienced when they were not given the foods. In one study, animals even preferred sugar over cocaine, as the former was a more powerful reinforcer of palatability and reward.[13]

As pharmaceutical companies develop medications (like Naltrexone) to address binge eating, food manufacturing companies are capitalizing on it by making their products even more addictive. This has led to the paradox of an industry promoting food addiction while another seeks to counteract it with medications. Most weight-loss drugs enhance feelings of fullness and reduce constant snacking urges, whereas the ultra-processed food industry aims to do the opposite—encouraging frequent snacking on foods that quickly absorb and diminish the sense of fullness. Both industries profit from human vulnerabilities. After fostering food addiction, the food industry sets the stage for the pharmaceutical sector to increase their profits with de-addiction drugs, creating a cycle of dependency.

Hacking Our Decision-Making Apparatus

The bond between food and me is like other relationships in my life: complicated, evolving, demanding, and in need of constant work.

—Ashley Graham

People addicted to food will continue to eat despite the negative consequences like weight gain, diabetes, depression or damaged relationships. Similar to compulsive gamblers and drug addicts, food addicts also have trouble resisting the temptation, even if they want to or have tried many times to cut back. However, this dependency doesn't happen overnight.

The science behind it is straightforward. Present a highly processed, appealing food item that generates a craving in consumers, prompting them to return for more. By exploiting the brain's reward centres, food companies establish a cycle where individuals become devoted customers of their manufactured products.

The brain is inherently driven to pursue rewards, and once triggered, this response leads to recurring behaviours. Whether it's sugar or cocaine, our neural pathways are drawn to stimuli that activate our reward centres, even if they are potentially addictive or harmful. The food industry has honed the art of captivating our senses and misleading us into consuming more than necessary. This all originated from comprehending how the brain guides decision-making processes.

The brain has numerous control centres that gauge the impulses and stimuli it receives, both from within and outside the body. It has thousands of switchboards for variables such as temperature, light, stress levels, morals, values, relationship thresholds and many environmental cues. All of these switchboards influence our brain's tiny control centres and enable us to react, respond and make decisions in response to different situations and stimuli. These switchboards are designed by evolution and work between the minimum and maximum set points, like a thermostat. This complex network contributes to the brain's adaptability and malleability.

These micro-control centres are designed to perform actions with three goals: looking around (to avoid pain and seek pleasure), eating and reproducing. It took millions of years of evolution for the human brain to fine-tune the output of these modules to be efficient. The success of the human race over other species is due to the efficient functioning of these modules. However, in recent years, our brains have been under tremendous pressure to adapt to situations and stimuli they have never been exposed to.

Evolution is a slow process. The rapid societal change makes it a struggle for our brains to keep up. The look around module is confronted with texting while driving. The eat module is exposed to highly processed foods and addictive junk food. The reproduction module is heavily influenced by virtual sex and pornography. The evolution of these three modules has not yet given the brain the chance to adjust and handle these strange behaviours healthily and productively.

This mismatch between social change and biological adaptation translates to numerous chronic under-the-carpet conditions that gradually escalate into debilitating disorders, such as chronic stress, mental illnesses, obesity and drug addiction.

Fast and Slow Brain Systems

The *Diagnostic and Statistical Manual of Mental Disorders* (DSM) describes addictions such as alcohol, cocaine, gambling, sex, etc. as behaviours tied to a specific substance or activity. However, addiction scientists agree that the brain pathways involved in almost all addictions are similar. Although genetic vulnerability adds to the risk of developing addiction, our behaviour and the environment we live in reinforce the habit.

Our brain operates on two levels: the fast brain and the slow brain.[14] The fast brain swiftly processes information and makes automatic, short-term decisions, with little involvement of willpower. Conversely, the slow brain system engages in long-term planning and conscious control. These systems have separate roles and operate in different contexts. A thriving brain depends on the effective interaction between them. There are situations where system one is more appropriate, and in other cases, system two is required. Often, their collaboration is essential to attain specific objectives.

System one, the fast brain, excels in straightforward scenarios, characterized by impulsivity. On the other hand, system two, the slow brain, comes into play for intricate or ambiguous tasks. It searches for rules in our surroundings, considers our values, ethics and other factors, making it a more time-consuming process. For instance, if you're stranded in a desert and come across organic matter, your fast brain instantly identifies it as food and prompts you to consume it—operating in survival mode. However, when you're at a well-stocked grocery store with various food choices, your slow brain engages, allowing you to deliberate on your decision.

When a person lets their fast brain take control, they run the risk of later regretting their impulsive decisions. Acting before their slow brain engages in a more deliberate decision-making process can lead to such regrets. This phenomenon helps explain why individuals sometimes consume an entire packet of cookies before even realizing they've started.

Emotional Eater's Brain

Our brain chemistry is surprisingly similar for all pleasurable activities, whether ecstasy while snorting cocaine, euphoria during orgasm or gratification while savouring a palatable meal. When specific centres in the brain called the pleasure centres are triggered, specific neurotransmitters are released. Genetic and environmental factors play a significant role in this process. What's more interesting is that our thoughts release neurotransmitters, which determine different actions. Every decision we make, every thought we entertain and every action we perform is influenced by the dance of chemicals in that tiny sliver of space between the synapses. The mere thought of palatable food releases specific chemicals at the synaptic junction, where hundreds of neurotransmitters determine our behaviour.

Dopamine is one such chemical. Every substance that is potentially addictive affects the dopamine transmitter system in the brain's reward centres. We now know that many foods also affect it.

Dopamine is a critical neurotransmitter because it affects three primary aspects of behaviour: attraction, avoidance and motivation. These three determine the dimensional sphere of our mental space—the dopamine system influences our vulnerabilities, tastes, preferences, dislikes and sense of purpose. Anything that affects our dopamine system will strongly affect these three areas of our lives. Any breakdown in this system will affect our decision-making capacity, sense of purpose and our ability to feel contented.

What happens when a person takes a hit of cocaine?[15] Cocaine molecules enter their bloodstream and attach to cell surfaces, blocking dopamine receptors and leading to a sudden surge in circulating dopamine molecules. This surge creates a rush and induces a feeling of being 'high'. With repeated cocaine use, the body adjusts to its continuous presence. It reduces dopamine receptors, causing less dopamine to bind (as the cocaine molecules have taken over). Consequently, the individual requires more cocaine to achieve the same previous high, a phenomenon known as drug tolerance.

Appetizing foods increase dopamine-mediated reward processing in the nucleus accumbens, the brain's pleasure centre, similar to an addictive drug.[16] When scientists removed these dopamine pathways experimentally, subjects showed decreased reward responses to palatable foods.

Dopamine and its receptors are involved in many essential life functions like emotions, motivation, cognition and reward systems in our brain. In a study conducted on tobacco smokers and past smokers, scientists discovered that ex-smokers could boost their dopamine receptors after quitting smoking.[17] Interestingly, studies conducted on obese individuals and those who lost weight through gastric bypass surgery produced results similar to smokers and ex-smokers—dopamine receptors bounced back after the individuals lost weight.

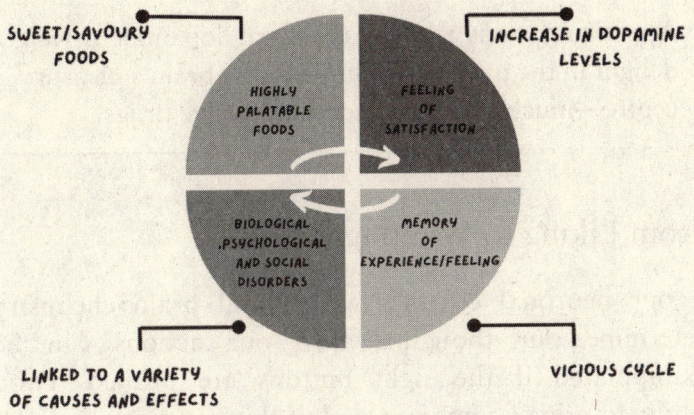

Figure 5.1: The Food Addiction Cycle

The way dopamine is managed in different parts of the brain—like the hippocampus and the amygdala— decides if someone becomes an emotional eater. Imagine feeling anxious and turning to food for comfort—your hippocampus kicks in, recalling the food's memory and providing comfort. This connection links comfort with food. When you eat that food, your dopamine reward system activates, reducing stress.

The striatum, a centre in the brain, affects decisions, motivation and how we perceive rewards.[18] Dopamine signalling in the striatum is linked to rewards, motivation and food intake, and it's also tied to drug-taking behaviour. Consuming palatable food triggers dopamine release, leading to a pleasurable feeling, much like with addictive substances.

Appetizing foods activate a burst of dopamine-driven delight in the nucleus accumbens, the brain's pleasure centre—much like the effect of addictive drugs.

From Liking to Wanting

If our neuronal circuit's wiring and brain chemistry determine our thoughts, then our actions can be manipulated if the right buttons are pushed. Food manufacturing companies exploit this system to make us eat their products compulsively.

The pleasurable effect elicited by an ingested substance, either food or recreational drug, is termed the 'liking response'. In 1996, scientists identified small regions in the brain called hedonic hotspots responsible for generating unconscious feelings of pleasure.[19] Apart from dopamine, other neurotransmitters such as opioids and Gamma-Aminobutyric Acid (GABA) work on these hotspots and amplify the pleasurable effects of certain types of food, thereby facilitating overeating. All individuals exhibit higher 'trait eating' behaviour depending on the taste elicited. Some are more sensitive to sweet tastes, others to salty ones. Preference is individual-specific and independent of hunger and caloric needs. If we know what tastes elicit a liking response to palatable foods, we can target particular snack foods specifically for these individuals.

These snack foods act as positive reinforcers with intrinsic properties to compel consumers to consume the food item repeatedly.[20] At this stage, the liking response turns into a 'wanting response', where the brain is sensitized to the reward cues from the repeated consumption of the palatable food.[21] Repeated exposure to the same reward becomes a conditioned and habit-forming behaviour. When individuals are sensitized to a particular snack item, they cannot stop eating it because this neuronal mechanism controls their thoughts and actions. This reinforcement of stimulus–reward association transforms voluntary behaviour into an automatic response. Snack manufacturers actively use all the latest science about transforming a liking response for a food item into a wanting response, resulting in a highly addicted consumer group.

From Wanting to Dependency

Tolerance and withdrawal are the two main characteristics of any addiction.[22] Substances of abuse initially activate the brain centres that elicit pleasurable emotional states such as euphoria, well-being or contentment. However, the brain then kicks in the counter-regulatory opponent processes that down-regulate this initial positive phase. With repeated cycles of excitatory and opponent processes, the body requires a higher stimulus level to feel the same excitement level. Consequently, a greater quantity and more frequent use of the previously rewarding substance is needed to maintain the same base level of contentment. This explains why statements like 'I need to eat more and more to get the feeling I wanted from eating fried onion rings' are not uncommon.

Even though individuals with food addiction don't exhibit 'physical' symptoms akin to drug withdrawal, they often experience irritability, mood swings, agitation, aggression and impulsivity when they abstain from eating. Without access to enjoyable food, they can experience negative emotional symptoms of withdrawal like impatience, anger, cravings and a sense of lacking. The term 'hangry', added to the Oxford English Dictionary in 2018, captures the heightened irritability during food abstinence. Fortunately, their symptoms and discomfort tend to ease when they have access to highly enjoyable food once more.

From Dependency to Compulsion

Compulsive behaviour is defined as an irresistible drive to participate in an intrusive behaviour that occurs outside one's control as a result of dysregulated mechanisms. Compulsive eating, characterized by excessive consumption of highly sugary and ultra-processed food, is no different. Brain scans of compulsive overeaters reflect similar brain changes as in drug addicts.

Researchers have classified compulsive eating behaviours into three forms: habitual overeating, overeating to relieve a negative emotional state and overeating despite adverse consequences.[23]

The uncontrollable eating behaviour observed in some overweight individuals has exactly the same characteristics of compulsivity as substance abuse disorders—one of the most notable features is that these individuals repeatedly engage in these harmful behaviours even in adversity. In this case, individuals continue to eat over and above their biological needs despite the physical and psychological health problems that stem from obesity.

The primary aspect of any addictive behaviour, be it gambling, recreational drug use or overeating, is a subjective feeling of losing control against the urge. Individuals can't break free from that behaviour, even when faced with the loss of relationships, debt, bankruptcy, illness, etc. Just as an individual continues to take drugs despite the consequences, some continue to overeat in spite of having medical conditions such as diabetes, high blood pressure, joint pain (due to excess fat mass) and low self-esteem, not to mention the pervasive stigma associated with being so vastly overweight.

Snack manufacturers are adept at harnessing the latest scientific understanding to convert a mere fondness for a delicious item into an irresistible craving. This clever manipulation creates a brainwashed and addictive group of consumers.

Genes, Leptin and Hyperphagia

Genetic defects in parts of the brain involved in controlling food consumption are the only cause of excessive eating not influenced by our social environment. Hyperphagia refers to overeating due to an abnormally strong hunger or desire to eat, resulting in an intense food-seeking behaviour that leads to aggression when food is denied.[24] It is thought to be associated with injury or lesions in the hypothalamus, a central feature of certain inherited genetic disorders, or due to certain genetic mutations. Hyperphagia frequently contributes to obesity. Recognizing that genetics are the root of its cause can provide immense value for anyone struggling with obesity.

The food reward hormone leptin also plays a significant role in overeating. Leptin is produced by fat cells, whose levels in the blood correlate with fat mass. Its function is simple but integral for our survival—to defend against starvation. Weight loss causes a drop in leptin levels in the blood, which causes changes in the body that help regain lost weight. How it achieves this feat is interesting. In a leptin-deficient state, food images trigger an intense activity in the brain's ventral striatum, an area highly concerned with pleasure and reward. This has been observed using a particular type of brain imaging called the functional MRI. For people with severe leptin deficiency, the sight, smell and even thought of food is profoundly effective mentally and physically. The end effects? Hyperphagia.[25]

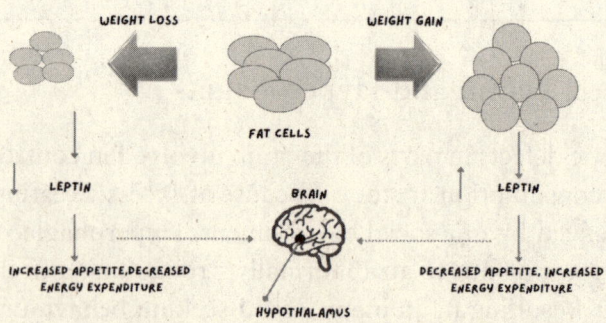

Figure 5.2: Leptin's Influence on Food Reward
and Overeating

Babies can be born with a leptin deficiency, which, if undiagnosed, leads to rapid and unexplained weight gain in the first few months of life, resulting in severe obesity.[26] The good news is that leptin injections can instantly treat and normalize hyperphagia within a week. Unless diagnosed and treated, a child with hyperphagia will almost certainly become a victim of obesity and, therefore, fat stigma—at home, in school and everywhere else they may go. Unfortunately, despite how treatable it is, treating or even detecting and diagnosing the condition is costly, meaning many victims don't receive life-changing help.

Understanding that genetic factors can lead to hyperphagia helps counter the belief that weight issues are entirely a person's fault. This awareness can support individuals in dealing with societal prejudices against people of any age who struggle with weight, addressing stereotypes like laziness and overeating.

* * *

'Food Is the Great Love of My Life'

When I am in trouble, eating is the only thing that consoles me. Indeed, anyone who knows me intimately will tell you, I refuse everything except food and drink. At the present moment, I am eating muffins because I am unhappy.

—*The Importance of Being Earnest*, Oscar Wilde

For most of us, our relationship with food is influenced by our parents and family who act as food providers, enforcers and role models since childhood. From the first years of life, we grow up in an adiposogenic environment which contributes to excess weight, yet our own people may be the first to shame us. We live in a social environment full of highly rewarding, inexpensive and easily accessible processed foods such as pastries, cakes, ice creams, sodas, chips, candies and various fast foods. Fatty, sugary and salty foods can cause neuroadaptation and behavioural changes comparable to those resulting from repeated use of cocaine, alcohol, nicotine and the like.

'Food is the great joy of my life,' wrote author Melanie Tait about her food addiction. 'I've sacrificed all else. It's taken precedence over partners, experiences, family, even my career. They don't believe I have a food addiction,' she says of her parents in a brutally honest and disturbing exposé. 'They believe I'm a weakling, incapable of self-control and a slacker.'[27]

Emotional distress or, more typically, boredom rather than hunger is the most prevalent trigger for eating. 'Fear dominated my life and I had dozens of resentments—I loathed everyone and everything,' an anonymous sufferer writes to addictiveeateranonymous.org, 'My days were spent alone at home, wallowing in self-pity (which I enjoyed), watching TV and eating.'[28] Chronic loneliness is so common that US Surgeon General Vivek Murthy declared that we are going through 'an epidemic of loneliness'.[29]

Exercising dietary restraint, or controlling our appetite, is a challenge in today's environment. Despite being aware of global nutritional guidelines, societal norms and pressures frequently interfere with our ability to regulate our eating. In developed countries, distinguishing between hunger and fullness cues is problematic. Our appetite is often influenced by personal food preferences, fixed meal schedules and social events, rather than genuine biological signals.

Our social interactions also play a massive role in hunger and satiety. For instance, it was discovered that we eat 35 per cent more when eating with a partner, 75 per cent more with three other persons and 96 per cent more with a group of seven or more. Even the ambiance might push us to eat more. We eat more in a room with brighter light, faster music and more colourful walls. In comparison, slow music makes us eat slower, lengthening the duration of our meals and giving us a better chance to tune in to our satiety cues. Whether we are eating fast or slow, most of us consume more food than our bodies need.

On foodaddiction.com, Emily described how her food addiction ultimately led to the termination of her career, 'At work, I always fell asleep at my desk and binged throughout the day, causing me to miss meetings. Food was taking over my life.'[30]

While we may not all be able to relate to Emily's adversity, most of us have overeaten to the point of feeling bloated. At some point, we had to unbutton our jeans and experienced clammy sweat, a racing pulse and a sluggish feeling after eating more than we required to satisfy our hunger. Even if we've done it occasionally perhaps during holidays or at a party, those who have a healthy connection with food are less likely to do it again. For someone with a food addiction, the dysfunctional satiety cues, leptin deficit, hyperphagia or binge eating disorder (BED) make the unpleasant sensation of overeating insufficient to prevent them from repeating the harmful activity. Bingeing, restricting, bingeing and restricting—this maladaptive cycle continues.

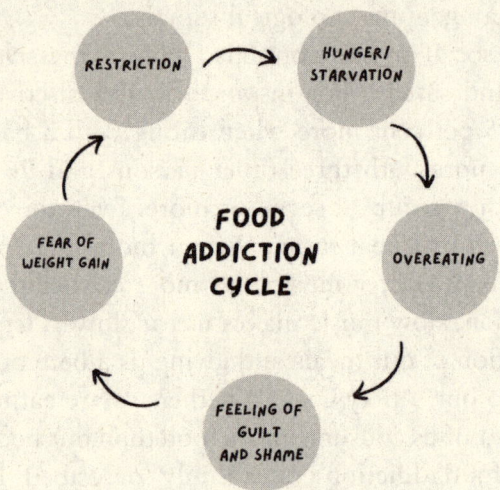

Figure 5.3: Food Addiction Cycle

Binge Eating Disorder vs Food Addiction[31]

After much contemplation, thirty-year-old Alice, with a BMI of thirty-two, decides to visit her doctor's office. She constantly thinks her eating may be out of control and doesn't know how to stop. At the doctor's, she explains, 'I often eat large amounts of food in one sitting, I feel a complete lack of control and I'm always detaching from myself during these times.' Pausing to take a deep breath, she continues, 'I eat alone in my room with the TV turned up loud to mask any sounds to hide from my roommate,' as she feels intense embarrassment and guilt. 'I have tried to stop for years, but I can't manage it.' At that first confession to her doctor, she felt defeated. Her self-esteem was at an all-time low, and she knew that she was suffering physically and mentally due to this behaviour.[32]

The distinction between binge eating and food addiction is important because appropriate treatment is dependent on a proper assessment of the root cause of the problem. The binge eating disorder (BED) was first noted by psychiatrist Albert Stunkard way back in 1959. In 1987, it was recognized as a feature of bulimia in the DSM. BED was only recognized as a disorder in its own right in the fifth edition of DSM in 2013, which was significant since it allowed people to access targeted treatment under their insurance plans and added legitimacy to the condition.[33] BED, the most common eating disorder in many countries, including India and the United States, is characterized by an individual's loss of control while eating, resulting in them bingeing on enormous amounts of food.

After an episode of binge eating, the individual often feels a great deal of guilt and shame, which is a big deterrent to seeking help. Binge eating affects both men and women at almost the same rate. Unlike bulimia patients, someone suffering from BED doesn't compensate for their food intake through fasting, purging, laxative abuse or over-exercising, meaning that they tend to gain a lot of weight and experience all of the side effects that come with obesity. Although obesity itself is not an eating disorder, it can be a consequence of one.

BED is mostly thought to be caused by a malfunctioning neurocircuitry in individuals with minimal influence from their environment. Most of the literature in this area is focused on treating the symptoms rather than discovering their root cause. The monster we are facing now, food addiction, is too big and we will not be able to successfully tackle it by managing its symptoms. We need to dive right into the root cause of the problem. Otherwise, we may be staring at more pills and procedures from drug manufacturers as our go-to tool to treat food addiction instead of addressing it holistically.

The term 'food addiction' was first introduced into the scientific literature in the 1950s.[34] A person is suffering from food addiction if he experiences frequent episodes of uncontrolled eating, followed by a feeling of distress and an inability to function normally as a result of overeating. We know 'too much' eating is a subjective experience, but in 2009, researchers Gearhardt, Corbin and Brownell of Yale University designed the Yale Food Addiction Scale (YFAS) to objectify the degree of food addiction.[35] Since then, it has become the most commonly used tool to measure food addiction.

> Recognizing the difference between binge eating and food addiction is important because choosing the right treatment relies on accurately identifying the underlying cause of the problem.

Moderation Is a Myth

We live in a social environment where food signals from TV advertisements, billboards and fast-food brands at restaurants, malls and grocery stores continually influence us. These cues hijack our eating habits, causing us to act automatically without conscious control.

There is rarely such a thing as moderation in this context, especially when it comes to highly refined food, due to its addictive potential and consumers' greater propensity to develop a tolerance for it. Refined food manufacturers know how difficult it is to consume their products in moderation. Yet, they choose to remain silent about it. When confronted, they tout that it's the individual's responsibility to consume in moderation and that their product is the perfect treat, balancing both enjoyment and health.

When suggesting a calorie-restricted diet for individuals dealing with excess weight, health coaches and dieticians need to keep in mind that those who have successfully cut down on calorie intake might already have the capacity to resist highly palatable foods. However, for most people, returning to old eating patterns becomes likely when the recommended diets lack the same tastiness and emotional comfort, ultimately leading them to fall back into compulsive eating habits.

> It is difficult to moderate the consumption of refined carbohydrate diets. They are intentionally designed to be addictive.

In her 2014 TedMed talk, neuroscientist Dr Nora Volkow, the director of the National Institute on Drug Abuse, observed, 'In all my years as a physician, I have never met a person who chose to be an addict, nor have

I ever met someone who chose to be obese. Imagine how frustrating it must be to be unable to stop doing something when you want to. Dismissing food addiction or obesity as self-control problems ignores the fact that for us to exert self-control, we require the proper function of the areas in our brain that regulate our behaviours.'[36]

The complexities of food addiction cannot be oversimplified, particularly because food is an essential necessity that cannot be easily avoided. While a heroin addict can choose to get clean and live without the drug, someone seeking recovery from food addiction cannot simply stop eating. We understand that it's unrealistic to ask a cocaine addict to have 'just a little bit' of the drug, yet we often expect those with food addiction to do so. Unlike other addictive substances, food cannot be completely eliminated from one's life. While an alcoholic can remove all alcohol from their surroundings and a smoker can stop buying cigarettes, a food addict must still navigate environments filled with their 'drug of choice'. They must make choices for their future well-being even when their present desires and cravings are strong. Recovery for a food addict occurs within a world where the substance harming them is also necessary for survival.

Any recommendation that involves a behavioural change to address food addiction must consider the role of the social environment and barriers to healthy eating. As much as we would like a simple solution to this problem, addressing food addiction is not merely asking a person to stop overeating. You need to equip the individuals with tools to build resilience in the face of the constant onslaught of food commercials and the appealing packaging of products that are only harming them. It requires educating people on how to fuel their bodies in the right way to feel full at the appropriate time while also feeling satisfied. You can ask someone to eat a green salad, but they are far more likely to reach for the cookie jar an hour later if they don't feel satisfied.

Medical professionals need to have as much information as possible on the circumstances surrounding an individual's overeating behaviour by including potential genetic and biological factors to build a complete picture of the situation and recommend treatments tailored explicitly for them. That is the only way to give each person the best chance of recovery from food addiction, overeating, binge eating and obesity.

> Advising a cocaine addict to consume only a small quantity of crack is absurd, yet we often impose a similar expectation on individuals with food addiction.

Putting It All Together

We are grappling with an intricate and multidimensional interplay of factors operating at various levels: the interplay of environmental and genetic elements on a macro scale, the interplay of social and evolutionary factors on a middle scale, and the interplay of molecular and synaptic dynamics on a micro level. Together, these components form a complex system of moving parts within the brain and body, influencing our decision-making, motivation, arousal, hunger, satisfaction, emotions, habituation and satiation. All of these elements contribute to the distinct behavioural patterns that individuals exhibit in their approach to food. Furthermore, the intricate web of chemical and hormonal signals within the brain adds an extra layer of complexity, making it a challenging puzzle for researchers to dissect and comprehend.

> Not feeling loved in your life? Allow yourself some chocolate. Sugar elicits love responses in our brain, making it addictive.

Clinical researchers and the food industry share a keen interest in identifying the substances within foods that possess a heightened potential for addiction. The food industry finds this concept intriguing as they can shape human behaviour by skilfully blending ingredients to create addictively appealing ultra-processed and mass-produced foods. Meanwhile, researchers recognize the importance of studying this area. If they can pinpoint foods with strong addictive potential, it might lead to policy recommendations such as labelling food packages with warnings like 'Caution: High Addiction Potential'. Such findings could also empower regulators to limit the availability of foods that contribute to the rising rates of obesity, diabetes and other metabolic disorders due to their addictive nature. Moreover, healthcare professionals could extend guidance to individuals grappling with food addiction, offering strategies to manage withdrawal symptoms, imparting knowledge about foods with addictive tendencies to avoid, and more.

The sooner such regulations come into effect, the sooner we can protect and help a whole new generation of people make wiser choices surrounding what they choose to consume. If we want to generate real, impactful change in our population, we need to inculcate the right attitude towards consuming the right foods from childhood because that's where our food addiction takes root.

Social pressures, the prevalence of inexpensive food, advertising influences, racial disparities, family customs and the domestic surroundings are just a few of the hindrances to achieving optimal nutrition. Our environment fosters addictive behaviours, contributing to a cycle of compulsive actions. If we consider food addiction akin to drug addiction, could it be worthwhile to establish food addiction programmes akin to those dedicated to drug addiction treatment?

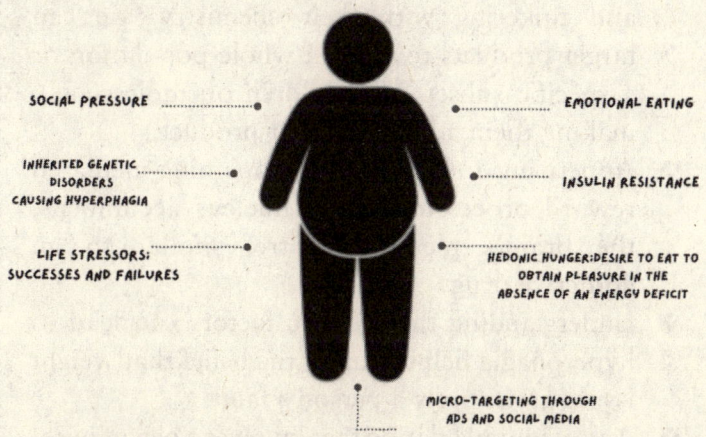

SOCIAL PRESSURE

INHERITED GENETIC DISORDERS CAUSING HYPERPHAGIA

LIFE STRESSORS: SUCCESSES AND FAILURES

EMOTIONAL EATING

INSULIN RESISTANCE

HEDONIC HUNGER:DESIRE TO EAT TO OBTAIN PLEASURE IN THE ABSENCE OF AN ENERGY DEFICIT

MICRO-TARGETING THROUGH ADS AND SOCIAL MEDIA

Figure 5.4: Factors influencing food addiction

Health educators must recommend an individualized diet plan to patients based on their behaviour and neurobiological traits. Engaging with a patient, developing a connection with them, empathizing with their situation, and assisting them in changing their behaviour and lifestyle for better results involves a different type of skill set than prescribing a pill or suggesting surgery.

At a Glance

❖ Many people who suffer from obesity also suffer from faulty satiety signalling in their brains.

❖ Our struggle to recognize when to cease eating arises because the foods we consume aren't inherently designed to signal when we're satisfied.

❖ By mixing and matching different threshold levels of substances, manipulating ingredients and tinkering with their chemistry, we can target products towards a whole population or a specific subset (like children or adolescents), making them addicted to our product.

❖ Appetizing foods increase dopamine-mediated reward processing in the nucleus accumbens, the brain's pleasure centre, similar to an addictive drug.

❖ Understanding that genetic factors can lead to hyperphagia helps counter the belief that weight issues are entirely a person's fault.

❖ Any recommendation that involves a behavioural change to address food addiction must consider the role of the social environment and barriers to healthy eating.

* * *

6

Flawed Nutrition Science Screwed Things Up for You

The association between refined carbohydrate and disease, and the fear that sugar may be injurious is as old as the written history of this sweet food. Denis Parson Burkitt, the late surgeon renowned for his work on cancer and nutrition, traced concerns surrounding sugar's nutritional value to India around 100 AD, soon after the cultivation and importation of sugar cane from New Guinea. Charake Samhita ascribed both obesity and diabetes to this 'new article of diet'.

—Proteins, Pathologies and Politics: Dietary Innovation and Disease from the Nineteenth Century

Nichole Barnum struggled with her weight for many years. After her first pregnancy, her weight soared significantly from just under 54 kg to over 80 kg. Even though she was able to reduce some of the weight, her weight further shot up to 98 kg after the birth of her second child. 'I would work out for an hour every morning. I jogged on the treadmill, used the elliptical, lifted weights, did squats and much more. IT WAS HARD. My weight slowly began to creep back up the moment I quit working out. Working out every day is not sustainable for me,' she lamented.

Nichole diligently counted calories, adhered to a rigorous 1800-calorie daily diet, and dedicated herself to seven days of weekly workouts, all without witnessing substantial results. Her spirits plummeted as she realized the entire regimen was unsustainable and her motivation dwindled. The effort felt like a fruitless endeavour, leaving her questioning the purpose of it all.

Over the last century, many weight-loss instructions have established a name for themselves, but the two most prominent ones, in particular, have significantly influenced the entire landscape of how our society views food and diets. They altered the fate of food policy and consequently, the eating patterns of millions of people across the world. Calorie counting and the low-fat diet are the two well-known weight-loss 'solutions', which are scientific distortions that have only exacerbated the problem of weight gain.

For decades, these two concepts have been sold to us. They hold some validity but only under certain conditions. In theory, these hypotheses found success in controlled laboratory environments, but they stumbled when applied to real individuals, in the real world.

Myth #1: Calorie Counting

A Calorie Is a Calorie[1]

We've all heard of a calorie—that mischief maker that gets higher the tastier something is. The number is supposed to tell us whether something is 'good food' or 'bad food'. When looking at a menu, some people will look at the calorie count even before looking at the price. High-calorie foods should be avoided, whereas low-calorie foods are lauded as healthy foods. Thousands of books, blogs and websites have shared how one can 'feel full with fewer calories', and several smartphone applications are now available to help us track and count the calories in everything we eat.

That's what we think calories are, but what *are* they?

French physicist and chemist Nicolas Clément (1779–1841) was the first person known to define and utilize the calorie as a unit of heat.[2] A calorie is a measurement of energy. It tells us how much heat is required to increase the temperature of a kilogram of water by one degree Celsius. It represents the amount of heat generated when a particular food is 'burned' in the body. Although we usually use the term 'calorie' solely in the context of food today, this term was unheard of in the field of human nutrition prior to the twentieth century. At that time, scientists calculated the heat generated by food using a calorimeter, a laboratory device used to measure the amount of energy produced or absorbed in a chemical reaction. However, measuring the heat value/energy value/caloric value of the same food when burned in the human body was inconceivable.

In 1780, chemist Antoine Lavoisier conducted an experiment using an ice calorimeter to explore how organisms release energy through metabolism and respiration.[3] He placed a guinea pig inside a container within another container filled with ice. He observed that the melting ice was directly related to the energy produced by the guinea pig. Interestingly, Lavoisier was also the first to suggest that nutrients played a crucial role in metabolism.

In 1827, an English physician named William Prout made a significant discovery. He found that a diet is made up of three main macronutrients: fat, protein and carbohydrates.[4] This concept was a significant discovery in the field of human nutrition and sparked enormous interest in the sector. As a result, various trials that altered nutritional thinking were carried out in laboratories across the West.

An American chemist, Wilbur Olin Atwater (1844–1907), conceived and developed the 'Atwater system' to measure the fuel value of macronutrients in units that became known as food calories.[5] The relationship between food intake and energy output could be measured using this system.

Atwater meticulously designed a special calorimeter, measuring 7 feet long, 4 feet wide and 6 feet tall. This chamber was made of copper, zinc and wood, and it was big enough for an adult to fit inside.[6] Atwater had a man in the room with a foldable cot, table and chair. As the man ate, drank, slept and did some light work, food and drinks were brought into the room and excreta was expelled. Atwater discovered that different types of food generated different amounts of energy. He concluded that the body digested different forms of food differently. He also discovered that any energy not used by the body's numerous metabolic processes was stored within the body. Atwater's findings were revolutionary at the time.

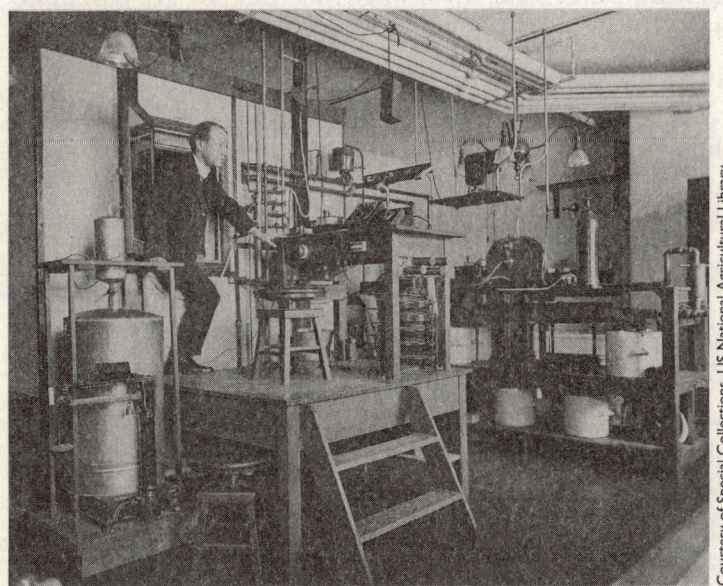

Figure 6.1: Subject exits respirator calorimeter in
Atwater's laboratory

According to the Atwater system, the caloric content of food is calculated by first determining the food's protein, carbohydrate and fat content, all measured in grams. The next step is to compute the number of calories in each macronutrient: 1g of protein and 1g of carbohydrate each generate 4 kilocalories of energy, while 1g of fat generates 9 kilocalories. Therefore, if a particular food item has 5g of protein, 10g of carbohydrate and 2g of fat, it contains: 5x4 + 10x4 + 2x9 = 20 + 40 + 18 = 78 calories. Hence, the total calories produced by burning (or digesting) that particular food within the body is 78 calories. Food manufacturers began using this system to calculate the calorie count to label their food packages, and it quickly became an industry standard.

Today, we don't have to work so hard to calculate the caloric content of the food we eat since a multitude of websites and apps are available to do it for us. For instance, the UK's NHS calculator can tell you the calorie count of 1,50,000 foods and drinks.

Being a biochemist, Atwater rightfully believed that a *calorie is a calorie* and that energy from any food source is reduced to the calories it generates when burned (digested), irrespective of the source from which it was obtained. Fifty calories from chocolate provide the same energy as fifty calories from carrots. However, it doesn't take much thought to figure out that Atwater's system was an extreme oversimplification of what happens to food once it enters the body and how much energy is generated from it. The type and quality of food, the amount of processing needed, its preservation, cooking, storage, the time of day the food is consumed, the digestion process and even the type of microbes living in your gut are some of the factors that affect how your body burns calories. This calorie counting concept does not consider how people burn different foods at different rates or how the method of cooking or preparing food can alter its absorption.

'A calorie is a calorie' reinforces the concept that the calorie is a sufficient way to describe the energy content of food.[7] One dietary calorie contains 4184 joules of energy, regardless of whether it comes from carbohydrates, proteins or fats. With this knowledge, it is easy to assume that all calories have equal quantitative value, but consider this: two fun-size bags of M&Ms and two hard-boiled eggs both contain about 140 calories. The eggs have protein and healthy fat that will keep you full for a longer duration, and are packed with vitamins and minerals. In contrast, M&Ms (colourful bite-sized candies) offer little nutritional value and are rich in refined sugar. This can lead to a quick surge and subsequent drop in blood sugar levels, causing you to crave another snack shortly afterwards. All calories are not created equal. Hence, careful calorie calculations don't always yield consistent results; you can eat the same number of calories as someone else yet have very different health outcomes.

Most people have been taught that losing weight is a matter of simple math. Cut 3500 calories and you'll lose a pound. However, experts have come to realize that this decades-old strategy is highly misguided.

A 2019 study published in *Cell Metabolism* by Dr Fatima Cody Stanford, an obesity specialist and assistant professor of medicine and paediatrics at Harvard Medical School, found that eating processed foods seems to provoke people to eat more refined snacks than natural foods.[8] In the study, twenty people split into two groups were offered meals with the same number of calories and similar amounts of sugar, sodium, fat, fibre and micronutrients, and were allowed to eat as much as they wanted. The key difference was that one group was given natural foods and the other, ultra-processed foods. After two weeks, the groups switched and ate the other diet for the next two weeks.

Dr Stanford observed that those who ate ultra-processed food gained weight faster. Furthermore, she noticed that participants who ate the processed foods ate 500 calories more each day on average, but when they ate the natural foods, their calorie intake decreased.

Calorie counting based on food labels provides an incomplete, sometimes inaccurate, picture of the food's actual nutritional and energy value. Though it is valuable to understand which foods are calorie-dense and which are lower in calories, it is a flawed methodology to base one's entire diet on calorie counting. Someone counting calories may choose to skip certain nutrient-dense foods because they are high in calories, such as avocados or walnuts, and instead choose something low in calories but equally low in nutritional value, such as a pack of potato chips. To add insult to injury, the accuracy of calorie counting from food labels based on the Atwater system is increasingly disputed. A 2012 study by a USDA scientist concluded that the measured energy content of a sample of almonds was 32 per cent lower than the estimated Atwater value.[9]

Furthermore, it is known that some calories are wasted without ever being chemically converted or stored. The idea of calorie-in and calorie-out to maintain a healthy weight is antiquated and just plain wrong.

Besides being imprecise and often ineffective on a physical and metabolic level, we must also consider the mental impact of minutely examining the caloric value of every little thing we eat. What starts as a strong-willed dedication can spiral into an insidious obsession for some.

Leslie Corona gives an account of her negative experience with counting calories.[10] After being overweight for most of her life, she was determined to attain an ideal weight of 66 kg. Hence, she got into the habit of calorie-restricted meals, exercising and using a calorie-counting app. This solid plan enabled her to reach her goal weight, but she couldn't stop despite achieving her goal. 'Something had automatically switched in my brain. I feared food. I could consume 1200 calories a day but was afraid to eat more because the thought of putting on weight terrified me. I didn't know how to maintain the number on the scale. I only knew how to lose it.' Besides tracking her calorie intake, she even began recording her calorie expenditure. 'I purchased a fitness tracker to be more accurate about my calorie burn. I'd walk for hours, clocking up as much as 60,000 steps every day. Then I started running since I discovered it was a more efficient technique of burning calories. Three miles became six, which became ten, then fourteen and then more. I'd run for hours at a time to log my activity minutes on my app and watch the calculator "grant" me more calories so I could eat.'

Predictably, Leslie's lifestyle was unsustainable and she snapped. After months of starving her body deeply, she began binge eating. 'I'd gobble down loaves of bread, quarts of ice cream and bags of granola in one sitting. I'd even eat spoons of raw coconut sugar. My gut felt like it was ready to burst, but I was determined to keep going.' Her bingeing and starvation cycle had been ongoing for over two years. Her eating obsession haunted her every waking hour. 'I was isolating myself to avoid food to the point where I hardly went to any family functions and events with friends. It's challenging to track foods without nutritional information, especially on meals you haven't prepared yourself.'

It got so bad that her fiancé threatened to cancel their wedding if she didn't seek professional help. Having been diagnosed with anxiety and a BED, she enrolled in an eating disorder programme, where her journey to recovery began. After a year of seeing various specialists, receiving help from the specialized programme and most importantly, deleting all her calorie and exercise tracking apps, Leslie is healthier.

Leslie commented that, for her, calorie counting 'became a dangerous obsession that turned into binge eating disorder'. Her experience is not unique. While calorie tracking can be an efficient technique for some people to manage their food intake and achieve their weight-loss objectives, it can also lead to an obsession for many people to the extent of self-isolation and withdrawal from social situations where calorie counting is challenging. In these cases, it is harmful to people's mental health and can significantly reduce the quality of their social lives. These are serious adverse effects that must not be overlooked.

Most people have been taught that losing weight is a matter of simple math. It turns out, this decades-old strategy is highly misguided.

Myth #2: The Low-Fat Diet

Incorrectly Linking High-Fat Diets with High Cholesterol

Scientific studies dating back to the 1940s revealed a potential connection between high-fat diets and elevated cholesterol levels. This led to the idea that reducing fat intake, particularly LDL or 'bad cholesterol', could help prevent heart disease. Ancel Keys, an American physiologist, further established the link between cholesterol and cardiovascular disease (CVD).[11] As more research supported the relationship between dietary cholesterol and CVD, the concept of adopting low-fat diets gained popularity for both heart disease prevention and weight loss among physicians and patients.

By the 1960s, the low-fat diet was touted to be suitable for high-risk heart patients and everyone else. After the 1980s, physicians, the federal government, the food businesses and popular health media supported the low-fat diet as an overarching ideology. Ironically, in the decades after the low-fat strategy gained ideological traction, Americans became fatter, culminating in today's obesity crisis. Nevertheless, the low-fat ideology held such a firm grip on the general public that any doubts or criticism were brushed aside.

Key's Nemesis: Yudkin

John Yudkin, a physiologist and nutritionist, was the first scientist to recognize the dangers of the low-fat diet and how it spurred people to consume more sugar daily.[12] In 1972, he published a book called *Pure, White and Deadly* to summarize the evidence that the overconsumption of sugar was a major health risk, more harmful than fat. He observed that its overconsumption led to a significant increase in obesity, diabetes, liver disease, gout, dyspepsia and some cancers. Half a century later, he was proven right on all counts.

'I hope that once you have read this book, I shall have convinced you that sugar is actually deadly,' Yudkin boldly declared in the concluding remarks of the opening chapter of his book *Pure, White and Deadly*. This statement drew strong opposition from the sugar industry and processed food manufacturers. In the last chapter of his book, Yudkin revealed efforts to undermine his research funding and block the publication of his work. He referenced Ancel Keys' use of harsh language and personal attacks to dismiss evidence suggesting that sugar, rather than fat, was responsible for numerous severe health issues.

Keys was hugely dismissive of Yudkin's work as it went against everything his research stood for.

Calorie Counting and the Low-Fat Diet Created a Flourishing Weight-Loss Industry

Starting from the 1960s, the prevailing calorie-counting doctrine, coupled with Ancel Keys' lipid-heart hypothesis, has wielded substantial influence over Western dietary policies. The weight-loss industry has been built on these two myths, with no success in sustainable and effective weight loss. This is evidenced by the soaring obesity rate over the past six decades. The food industry heavily promoted calorie counting to the point where the world began to rally around the concept. Unfortunately, many of these diets are nothing but marketing strategies, backed by biased and misapplied science, targeted towards vulnerable and gullible individuals.

Any chef will tell you that fats add flavour and texture to the cooked food, whereas carbs pack a significant satiation punch. But when ultra-processed food makers wanted to remove fat without losing its palatability, intensifying refined carbs was the obvious solution. In the name of a low-fat diet, healthy fats were substituted with refined carbs. This swap became the main culprit behind the rising rates of insulin resistance, diabetes and obesity. A 2014 study by the Environmental Working Group found that the average low-fat breakfast cereal contains nearly 25 per cent sugar by weight.[13] We've been conditioned to believe that low-fat or non-fat yogurt is a healthy food suitable for weight loss, but 8 ounces of fruit-flavoured, non-fat yogurt contains 47 grams of sugar, nearly twelve teaspoons.

Fats play a vital role as essential nutrients, providing significant energy for our bodies and holding a crucial place in our diet. They facilitate nutrient absorption, contribute to healthy skin and hair, regulate body temperature, strengthen our immune system, and provide insulation to internal organs. Moreover, fats influence hormonal reactions, particularly the way our bodies respond to insulin. When fat intake is too low, it can result in dry and brittle hair and skin, while also increasing the risk of malnourishment due to poor nutrient absorption. Furthermore, low-fat products often contain high levels of refined carbohydrates, which can lead to insulin resistance, potentially causing diabetes and obesity.

Food manufacturers and marketing gurus invest millions every year touting low-fat products as the answer to obesity and the key to a healthy diet, thereby ingraining such beliefs in us and forcing millions of people to opt for the low-fat option of their favourite bread, cereals, dairy products and soft drinks. Despite their promises to aid in weight loss, the obesity rates are rising in tandem with the rise in popularity of the low-fat diet.

Besides being supported by the sugar industry-funded research, organizations often use renowned celebrities to sell their low-fat products. For example, Pepsi has been endorsed by musicians such as Beyoncé, Britney Spears, Christina Aguilera, Enrique Iglesias, Justin Timberlake, Katy Perry, Mariah Carey, Calvin Harris, Nicki Minaj, One Direction, Shakira and will.i.am, and athletes such as Lionel Messi, Saquon Barkley, David Beckham and Bradley Beal, as well as influencers like Kendall Jenner, appealing to a large number of susceptible consumers.

In this landscape, how can anyone maintain a healthy weight? How can people ever free themselves from the mass media influence?

Since the 1960s, the calorie-counting dogma, paired with the lipid-heart hypothesis of Ancel Keys, has significantly influenced the dietary policy in the West.

How the Industry Misuses Science . . . to Its Advantage

The year 1967 stands as a significant moment in medical history, marking two pivotal developments—one for the better and one for the worse.

In that year, Christiaan Bernard, a skilled surgeon from Cape Town, South Africa, performed the world's inaugural human-to-human heart transplant at Groote Schuur Hospital, a monumental advancement in medicine.[14] Concurrently, the landscape saw a different shift, with numerous sugar companies beginning to invest in Harvard University labs to sponsor research promoting refined sugar as a healthier substitute for dietary fats.[15]

The research results were published in the *New England Journal of Medicine* in 1967, although the substantial funding from the sugar industry behind the study was not disclosed.[16] The study's conclusion advocated the reduction of fat and an increase in sugar consumption to combat heart disease. Capitalizing on this, the sugar industry heavily marketed the concept, using medical research to endorse their low-fat, high-carb diet approach. This marked the inception of the sugar industry's influence on medical research and their manipulation of the debate in their favour.

These misleading research findings propagated by the sugar industry led the public to embrace the idea of consuming substantial quantities of sugar as normal.[17] The mantra of 'calories in, calories out' implied that you could burn off excess sugar calories by simply visiting the gym. Meanwhile, the idea of consuming less sugar and fat, and prioritizing vegetables and wholefoods, was met with resistance among the American population. Many considered this dietary shift impractical and unsustainable.

Regrettably, the disturbing reality persists: the act of intentionally skewing data or manipulating research methodologies in the realm of medical studies continues to occur even today. This was highlighted by nutrition professor Marion Nestle in a 2016 *New York Times* article.[18] In the article, Nestle revealed the dubious influence behind a review published in the *Annals of Internal Medicine*, which sought to discredit warnings about excessive sugar consumption. The study boldly asserted that the cautions against sugar overindulgence were based on 'weak evidence' that was unreliable. Notably, the study was financially backed by multinational food and agrochemical corporations.

Predictably, these deliberate efforts to manipulate study outcomes in favour of the food industry have significantly contributed to the global burden of obesity.

Nutritional Policies: Are They a Part of the Solution or a Part of the Problem?

In 1973, Richard Nixon, the thirty-seventh US President, strategically employed food restrictions to gain a political edge over his opponents.[19] This tactic was set in motion in 1971 when Nixon was seeking re-election. While the Vietnam War was eroding his domestic support, escalating food prices also posed a significant concern among voters. To bolster his chances of securing another term, Nixon needed to reduce food costs, which necessitated placating a powerful lobbying group—farmers. In pursuit of a solution, Nixon enlisted the help of Earl Butz, a scholar hailing from Indiana's agricultural hub. Butz, an agricultural scientist, came forward with an audacious proposal to reshape the public's dietary choices.

Butz enticed farmers to massively increase the production of a more economical crop—corn. This surge in corn cultivation led to livestock gaining weight across the United States. Burgers became larger and fries cooked in corn oil packed on extra ounces. Even chickens that feasted on corn saw their size swell significantly.

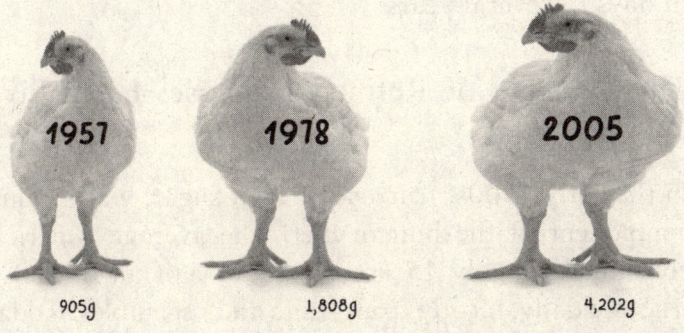

905g   1,808g   4,202g

Figure 6.2: Change in Chicken size since the 1960s

Due to the surplus of corn, it became an affordable food choice widely accessible in American stores. Corn found its way into nearly every type of cuisine, making appearances in cereals, cookies, flour, spreads, sauces and a wide range of processed foods.

However, by the mid-1970s, corn was becoming scarce. To address this issue, Butz took a trip to Japan and stumbled upon a game-changing scientific development: the large-scale production of high fructose corn syrup (HFCS), also known as glucose-fructose syrup in the UK.[20] This thick, delightful syrup was derived from surplus corn and proved incredibly cost-effective. While refined fructose in the form of HFCS was discovered in the 1950s, it wasn't until the 1970s that an industrial manufacturing process was developed to harness it. HFCS quickly found its way into countless products, enhancing sweetness and extending the shelf life of various items from a matter of days to several years.

The Dangers of Refined Fructose: Fatty Liver and Beyond

In the early 1900s, fructose or fruit sugar, was a minor component of the human diet. The average American consumed roughly 15 grams (about half an ounce) of fructose daily, mostly from fruits and vegetables. Today, we consume four to five times that amount, almost entirely from refined sugars found in breakfast cereals, pastries, sodas, fruit drinks, and other sweet foods and beverages.

The human body handles glucose and fructose, the two most common sugars in our diet, in distinct ways. While almost every cell can utilize glucose for energy, only liver cells can metabolize fructose for energy. However, how the liver processes fructose, especially when there's an excess of it in the diet, could pose potential risks to the liver, arteries and heart.

From Fructose to Fat

Upon entering the liver, fructose sets off a series of intricate chemical reactions. Through a process called lipogenesis, the liver transforms fructose, a carbohydrate, into fat. When there's an abundance of fructose, minuscule fat droplets start to gather within liver cells. This accumulation is termed non-alcoholic fatty liver disease (NAFLD), as it mirrors the effects seen in the livers of individuals who excessively consume alcohol.

Before 1980, NAFLD was almost unknown. Today, it has been on the rise globally, including in India. It's estimated that up to 30 per cent of the Indian population may be affected by NAFLD. Between 70 per cent and 90 per cent of people with obesity or diabetes are also diagnosed with NAFLD.

If identified in its early stages, NAFLD can be reversed. But if ignored, it can progress, leading to mild damage known as non-alcoholic steatohepatitis (*steato* meaning fat, and hepatitis meaning liver inflammation). If this inflammation worsens, it can advance into cirrhosis, a serious outcome marked by the build-up of scar tissue and eventual loss of liver function, which can be life-threatening.

Beyond the Liver

Excess fructose breakdown in the liver not only leads to fat accumulation but also:

- raises triglycerides
- increases harmful LDL cholesterol (often called bad cholesterol)
- encourages visceral fat build-up around abdominal organs
- raises blood pressure
- leads to insulin-resistant tissues
- produces more harmful free radicals that can damage DNA and cells

According to a Framingham Heart Study report, NAFLD is related to metabolic syndrome, an assortment of cellular aberrations that significantly increase the risk of heart disease. Other studies have linked fructose intake to high blood pressure.[21] However, many experts in the food industry are unwilling to confirm a clear link between fructose and NAFLD, obesity, diabetes and heart disease.

Although higher intakes of fructose are associated with many diseases, it is difficult to design clinical trials to prove the causation. Moreover, dozens of articles counter every research that links high fructose intake to metabolic diseases.

A 2009 article titled 'Misconceptions about High-Fructose Corn Syrup: Is It Uniquely Responsible for Obesity, Reactive Dicarbonyl Compounds, and Advanced Glycation End Products?' appeared in the *Journal of Nutrition* and was authored by John S. White, a consultant to the food and beverage industry specializing in nutritive sweeteners.[22] His clients included food industry councils, trade organizations and individual companies.

White strongly advocated for HFCS in food, promoting its innocence in the development of metabolic diseases like diabetes and obesity. While his article rightly acknowledged that HFCS was not the sole contributor to the obesity burden, it also downplayed the negative effects of sugar on health. The challenge extends beyond HFCS or highly processed foods, encompassing the addictive nature, affordability and appeal of foods that have driven consumption of larger portions, with frequent snacking becoming the norm.

The presence of hidden sugar in the foods we eat every day, coupled with the food industry lobbying to influence policies governing the manufacturing and distribution of such high-sugar products, makes it nearly impossible to limit or control the amount of sugar we consume.

The rise in adiposity and the struggle to maintain a healthy weight have paralleled the industrialization of ultra-refined food products, notably refined corn, soy and wheat.[23] These foods can be formulated to trigger addictive behaviours, fostering a lifetime of consumption for mass-producing food manufacturers. The adoption of widespread dietary guidelines based on flawed science further compounds the issue. Despite recent updates, the iconic food pyramid, introduced in 1992 to classify foods by health and nutritional value, remains ingrained in the minds of both medical professionals and the public. The advice emphasized reducing fat and oil intake while increasing consumption of carbohydrates like cereals, rice, pasta, bread, etc.

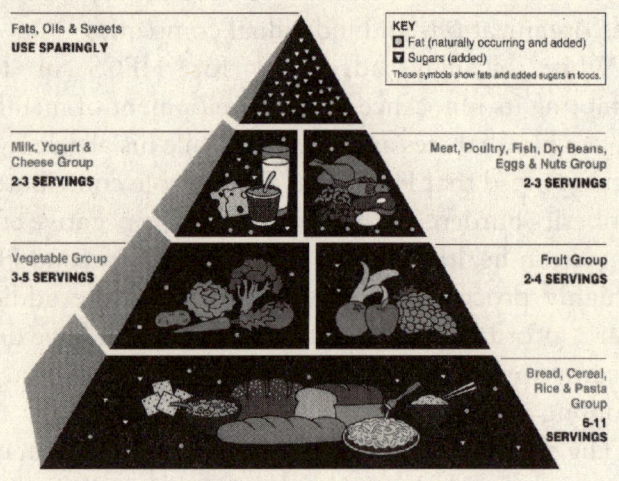

Figure 6.3: The USDA's original food pyramid, from 1992 to 2005[24]

The Problem With Universal Dietary Guidelines

The USDA has been issuing dietary guidelines since 1894, the first of which was written by Atwater. Since 1980, the USDA and the US Department of Health and Human Services (HHS), have published the 'Dietary Guidelines for Americans'. These guidelines, released every five years, provide the basis for federal food and nutrition policies as well as nutrition education initiatives for the public and healthcare professionals. This is accomplished in two steps: first, the most relevant nutrition-related public health issues and dietary strategies are identified; and second, effective communication messages are formulated to educate the public and change their behaviour.

Since its inception, the 'Dietary Guidelines for Americans' has seen many revisions based on population and sub-population research. The problem with such universal recommendations is that the data from population studies provide answers only pertinent to the average population. These studies are designed to develop standardized guidelines and public health policy and consequently, do not tell us whether the recommendations work at an individual level. Although done with the right intentions, the single biggest mistake we as nutritionists and healthcare professionals make is taking these universal dietary guidelines and applying them to individuals. By doing so, we overlook the fact that all individuals are a unique mix of genetics, environment and lifestyle.

If one diet works for a friend or family member, it might or might not work for us. In truth, we will never find a simple universal solution that works for everyone. What we require is personalized care specifically tailored to tackle the health issues we encounter.

* * *

Science Is a Double-Edged Sword

How do you entice the citizens of the world's most advanced country, the US, to consume an average of 32 kg of refined sugar, 90 grams of salt and a staggering 15 kg of cheese each year? The secret lies in a cleverly orchestrated and closely guarded strategy deftly executed by the processed food industry.

Zohnerism and the Art of Tactful Communication

In 1997, Nathan Zohner, a fourteen-year-old student at Eagle Rock Junior High School in Idaho Falls, Idaho, took centre stage with a science fair project titled 'How gullible are we?' He decided to petition for a ban on using hazardous substances in everyday life, with his focus being on a particular chemical: dihydrogen monoxide. During his presentation, Zohner provided scientifically sound arguments to his classmates about why this substance should be banned. He pointed out that dihydrogen monoxide:

- Causes severe burns in its gaseous state
- Corrodes and rusts metal
- Contributes to numerous deaths each year
- Is present in things like tumours and acid rain
- Can lead to excessive urination and bloating if ingested

Science Is a Double-Edged Sword

How do you entice the citizens of the world's most advanced country, the US, to consume an average of 32 kg of refined sugar, 90 grams of salt and a staggering 15 kg of cheese each year? The secret lies in a cleverly orchestrated and closely guarded strategy deftly executed by the processed food industry.

Zohnerism and the Art of Tactful Communication

In 1997, Nathan Zohner, a fourteen-year-old student at Eagle Rock Junior High School in Idaho Falls, Idaho, took centre stage with a science fair project titled 'How gullible are we?' He decided to petition for a ban on using hazardous substances in everyday life, with his focus being on a particular chemical: dihydrogen monoxide. During his presentation, Zohner provided scientifically sound arguments to his classmates about why this substance should be banned. He pointed out that dihydrogen monoxide:

- Causes severe burns in its gaseous state
- Corrodes and rusts metal
- Contributes to numerous deaths each year
- Is present in things like tumours and acid rain
- Can lead to excessive urination and bloating if ingested

considered fraud or corruption, these institutions are flawed in ways that harm the health of millions.

The manipulation of science by the industry takes various forms. By overly highlighting the importance of exercise in weight loss, they manage to promote a range of items like snacks, drinks, shakes and high-tech exercise gear under the guise of 'health'. These sales thrive thanks to the idea of a low-calorie diet and a flourishing fitness industry, backed by scientific research and endorsements from celebrities funded by the food industry.

Anyone attempting to lose weight in our society faces an uphill battle. The diets created for our nourishment make us unhealthy and are one of the many pitfalls we encounter. As they struggle to lose weight in impossible circumstances, people are also burdened by the stigma that comes with their weight, compounded by the guilt they feel for doing all they are told to do and still not seeing any results.

* * *

At a Glance

❖ 'A calorie is a calorie' is problem #1. It reinforces the concept that a 'calorie' is a sufficient way to describe the energy content of food. Calorie counting provides an incomplete, sometimes inaccurate, picture of a food's actual nutritional and energy value.

❖ The low-fat diet hypothesis is problem #2. It has led to the replacement of fat with refined sugar and processed carbs, both of which we know are addictive and strongly linked to obesity and obesity-related illnesses.

7

Your Willpower Can Be Easily Hacked

To predict the impact of an advertisement or a product based on neurological predispositions and real-time brain activities is the purpose of the field of 'Consumer Neuroscience' or, in simple terms, 'Neuromarketing'.

—Abhijit Naskar

During a mid-year parent–teacher meeting, Jonas's head teacher approached his mother and expressed concern about his weight. Though she hadn't given much regard to his weight, Jonas's mother scheduled a visit to his paediatrician the following week. While waiting at the reception, she glanced at her fourteen-year-old son. He was larger than most children and was constantly compared to other boys his age. In his family, all men were tall. Jonas was tall too, but with a touch of chubby, *but that's just puppy fat*, she thought to herself. As they waited, he played a game on his phone while snacking on a bag of chips. *A small bag isn't unreasonable for a growing boy who requires sustenance, is it?* Suddenly, Jonas burst out laughing at something on the screen as he watched. He was a happy, courteous and friendly youngster who had a lot of friends.

When they entered the office, the doctor requested Jonas to stand on the weighing scale and proceeded to measure his blood pressure. Upon keying the data into the computer, the doctor asked them to share their general daily routine to understand Jonas's lifestyle more closely. His mother stated that Jonas spent three to four hours on the TV/iPad daily, snacked regularly between meals and drank a soda with most meals, and also had a couple of in-between meals (*kids have to stay hydrated, right?*). Jonas didn't have any pre-existing health concerns and at 5'7", he weighed 95 kg. The doctor recommended some blood tests and referred them to a dietician specializing in adolescent obesity. Jonas and his mom left the room perplexed. The young man was upset—he had always been proud of his size as it made him appear strong on the football field and his family had always told him what a big, strong young man he was. His mother couldn't bear to see him so upset, so on the way home, she decided to stop and treat him to a burger and a milkshake.

Food Marketing to Children and Teens

Today, obesity affects approximately 20 per cent of children aged two to seventeen, nearly triple the rate in the 1970s.[1] Metabolic syndrome, sleep apnea, acid reflux, pseudotumour cerebri[2] (Increased intracranial pressure) causing incessant headaches and inability to focus, high blood pressure, early-onset diabetes, PCOS in young girls, psychiatric illnesses such as depression and eating disorders, are just a few of the problematic consequences of childhood obesity, apart from the emotional burden that children and adolescents gradually learn to bear due to their larger bodies.

Childhood and teenage obesity disproportionately impact lower and middle-income groups due to the elevated cost of nutritious foods. The primary contributor is an imbalanced diet rich in sugary beverages and highly processed foods. Beyond the financial barrier posed by healthier options, young individuals are also susceptible to developing an addiction to and dependence on these lower-quality food choices.

Advertising Targets the Vulnerable

As adults, we can recognize buzzwords such as 'low-fat', 'high protein' and 'superfood' when they appear on our screens. The youth, on the other hand, are an easy target— they are arguably the most susceptible to being persuaded by such advertisements because they are oblivious to huge corporations' targeted promotional techniques. Other ads target vulnerable parents, for example, the Wonder Bread ads.[3] The ad claims that the bread is a good source of calcium (which it is) and can help enhance memory (which is entirely unproven) to target parents who have minimal knowledge about nutrition and are simply trying to give their children the best.

The advertising and marketing of food products significantly influence food choices, especially among young people. Food preferences established from an early age and maintained into adulthood create a foundation for long-term health consequences for an individual. Young children who are obese are more likely to grow into obese adults, putting them at a higher risk of heart disease, stroke, cancers and other illnesses related to adiposity. In a report from the World Cancer Research Fund (WCRF), a study revealed that children exposed to just 4.4 per cent of food advertising are likely to consume up to sixty extra calories worth of junk food a day.[4]

Thanks to artificial intelligence's algorithm-based marketing, exposure to marketing and advertisements has become highly efficient. As of 2016, children aged 2–14 see an average of ten to eleven television commercials per day, amounting to approximately 4000 ads per year.[5] These are just television commercials. What about the advertisements on other platforms such as internet promotions, product placements, celebrity endorsements flooding social media, digital and print magazines, billboards, video games and even the logos on school vending machines? The food industry spends the most money advertising fast foods, carbonated beverages and breakfast cereals every year, which are the products that appeal directly to young people.

In 1980, the US Federal Trade Commission's authority to restrict food advertising was dismissed by Congress due to corporate lobbying.[6] Another attempt to restrict was made with bipartisan legislation in 2009 by creating the Interagency Working Group on food marketing to children between ages 2–17. However, pushback from organizations like the Grocery Manufacturer's Association and claims that the recommendations were 'unworkable' sabotaged its success in curbing advertising and marketing aimed at children. Today, national programmes such as Healthy Eating Research oversee responsible food marketing to children. However, they fail to make a dent in the frequency of such advertising due to heavy corporate lobbying from the food and beverage industry. In 2018 alone, the industry spent $29 billion to continue advertising to this vulnerable yet lucrative market.[7]

We hear these lobby groups ring out as far as the halls of Congress. In 2005, one US Congressman argued, 'The Personal Responsibility in Food Consumption Act, or the Cheeseburger Bill, is about self-responsibility. If you overeat, you get fat. It is your fault. Don't try to blame somebody else.'[8] This bill aimed to prevent legislative and regulatory functions from being usurped by civil liability actions against food manufacturers, marketers, distributors, advertisers, sellers and trade associations for claims of injury relating to a person's weight gain, obesity or any health condition associated with weight gain or obesity. In simple terms, the bill prevented anyone from taking legal action against the food industry for contributing to their obesity. It was a gag on obesity-related litigation.

The idea of preventing frivolous lawsuits against food industry giants such as McDonald's essentially closes the doors of courthouses to anyone seeking to question the causal relationship between fast foods and obesity.

We are all indeed responsible for what we eat, but that doesn't mean we have no right to question where our food comes from and what ingredients are in it. For instance, we now recognize how addictive nicotine is and the health risks associated with smoking, and we no longer see cigarette advertisements on our televisions. Marlboro and Benson & Hedges no longer sponsor sports teams, and we don't see people smoking in television shows and children's movies.

It's little wonder that research continuously proves strong associations between advertising of non-nutritious foods and rates of childhood obesity.[9] However, limiting screen time is a titanic task for parents, who are highly influenced by the exploitative advertising of processed food industries. It is nearly impossible to restrict access to billboards and general published advertising in our world today. Parents and children alike are victims of the society we have created.

> We are all indeed responsible for what we eat, but that doesn't mean we have no right to question where our food comes from and what ingredients are in it.

The Society of Our Making

Science, pop culture, globalization and religion are the four major factors impacting our lives. They rely on marketing to promote their products, services or doctrines. Marketing and advertising have been practised since the dawn of civilization, but the turn of the twentieth century witnessed the emergence of a new form of marketing that proved to be intrusive, slick and calculated.

The post-world war era saw not just the first substantial economic boom but also a considerable shift in marketing and advertising practices. Travelling salesmen successfully advertised and sold their products despite a lower disposable income. Around the year 1900, roughly 3,50,000 travelling salesmen in the United States sold goods directly to consumers by advertising their products in public or on street corners.[10] Unlike the current ads, early print advertisements had no eye-catching graphics and consisted solely of text. Soon, dazzling graphics and canny slogans edged out wordy product descriptions and pushy salesman. One such ad was Kodak's 'You press the button . . . we do the rest' campaign of 1891.[11]

By the 1920s, advertising was already popular and it significantly shifted consumer habits. Edward Bernays, an American business consultant and Sigmund Freud's nephew, was primarily considered the pioneer of the modern public relations (PR) industry. He redefined the status quo by instilling behavioural psychology and scientific methods into marketing and advertising, producing 'the engineering of consent'.[12]

Bernays used this strategy to appeal to the subconscious mind and manipulate consumers' will. In the 1920s, an American Tobacco Company approached Bernays about their cigarette brand, Lucky Strike.[13] While smoking had gained some popularity among women during World War I, it was still regarded as improper for a woman to smoke, particularly in public. Under Bernays' recommendation, Lucky Strike sought to capitalize on the women's suffrage movement and their emerging sense of freedom across the United States in the wake of the war. Bernays reframed cigarettes as a shortcut to a slimmer waistline and a tool for equality. He created ads featuring famous, attractive and fashionable American women smoking publicly. In a carefully crafted PR move, women interviewed afterwards referred to cigarettes as their 'torches of freedom', lighting the way to the day when women would smoke on the street as casually as men. The campaign was a huge success. The percentage of women who smoked more than tripled from 5 per cent in 1923 to 18.1 per cent in 1935.

'It's like opening a gold mine in front of our yards,' said J.B. Duke, president of the American Tobacco Company, in response to the cash generated by selling cigarettes to women. Duke's 'torches of freedom' ultimately established the cigarette as a symbol of both freedom and equality for women. The marketing was so successful that it was included in the rations given to the US combat troops during World War II. In the 1930s and 1940s, Lucky Strike was the best-selling cigarette brand in the United States.

World War II resulted in a surplus of goods produced by American companies, while demand remained constant. The excess goods were sold based on rational factors such as durability and value. However, according to Freud, people generally make decisions based on emotion rather than reason. As a pioneer in studying the mind, he conceptualized the subconscious as highly impressionistic and instrumental in people's decision-making processes. The Freudian psychoanalytical theory became the saving grace for advertising agencies to mass-market their surplus goods. Big industries took note and rapidly realized that emotional desire can be fuelled through effective marketing by hampering rational thought.

Bernays applied Freudian psychology by employing behaviourism in advertising the Beech-Nut Packing Company, which was experiencing difficulty in selling its bacon. Bernays pressed his company's internal physician to support his stand that one should eat a big breakfast rather than a light one. The same physician wrote to 5000 doctors across the country in a bid to affirm the benefits of having a hearty breakfast and 90 per cent agreed. This study was widely publicized, with headlines such as '4,500 Physicians Urge Heavy Breakfasts to Improve American People's Health'.[14] These publications explained to the public that bacon and eggs should be included in any diet, which resulted in widespread consumption of bacon for breakfast across America in an enduring marketing win.

Bernays viewed individuals as part of a broader social organism and said, 'Touch a nerve at a sensitive spot and you get an automatic response from specific members of the organism.' Through his approach, he influenced the lifestyle habits of Americans and the standard code of conduct for the new PR industry. Scaremongering and anxiety-inducing tactics began to be used to peddle non-essential products, many of which had adverse health effects, in a trend that we still see. In reality, we are sold not only on what we gain from a product but also on what we lose without it.

Today, ad companies use psychographic attributes of individuals and communities with complete profiles of individuals constructed based on their interests, attitudes, values and behaviours. An individual's profile is meticulously created using sophisticated artificial intelligence algorithms, which is then used to follow consumers from morning to night, from buses to billboards, television, radio, social media platforms, websites and smartphones.

When it comes to our eating and lifestyle choices, we are not consciously choosing but rather being targeted and coerced into adopting habits by PR companies. By preying on people's fears, weaknesses and emotions, many American businesses systematically transformed citizens into consumers—whether they needed a product or not. Furthermore, a vast number of advertisements are targeted towards children. Sugary cereals, candies and soft drinks are geared towards an audience that will carry the brand into their adult lives.

By preying on people's emotions, many corporations systematically transformed citizens into consumers— regardless of the actual need for the products.

Advertising is all about communication and persuasion. After manufacturers prepare a product for the marketplace, they need to raise awareness about their product and persuade people to buy it. Usually, many manufacturers compete in the market to sell their product and the competition is stiff, especially if it is a food item. All manufacturers spend a great deal of money on advertisements to inform people about their products and influence people's behaviour and actions. In the process of selling, they use various means to validate their claim. The interesting part is that the manufacturers figured out that they could create a need where there previously was none, through advertisement. For example, by adding a style element, the need for a particular dress can be made; by adding an emotion, the demand can be created for any product. The more intensely you can convince consumers to purchase your product, the more successful you are in the market.

Advertising invades our minds—it aims to make people want a particular product, regardless of whether or not they need it. In the twentieth century, advertising was considered one of the most influential institutions in America. By the mid-century, the country was spending more on advertising than on education or farming.

A common tactic employed by marketing agencies is to omit any educational or informative material about the product. Instead, they appeal directly to the emotional urges of the consumer and promise us something that is hard to resist.

Our diamond ring will ensure that you and the woman of your dreams will live happily ever after.

Your grandchildren will love you more if you give them our chocolate.

Our car is the safest if you want the best for your family.

For the holiday of a lifetime, book with us.

For the kitchen of your dreams, choose us.

The Fallacy of Free Will

Modern society is built upon the notion of free will as the keystone of civilized life. Regardless of a person's circumstances, an individual is 'free' to make decisions after carefully considering the pros and cons based on available information. However, many pre-existing social conditions shape the world we are born into. These conditions determine how factors such as race, gender, financial status, religion and others will shape our lives to limit our so-called free will, rendering it no more than an ideology.

This emphasis on free will and individuality has led to the belief that nobody but you are responsible for what happens to you. You have used your best judgement in any given situation. This belief has led to the stigma surrounding obesity, perpetuating the idea that fat people are fat because of their bad actions and poor choices, leading to feelings of guilt, shame and helplessness.[15]

Our progressive society reinforces the idea that we determine our fate. Neuroscientists and philosophers have been extensively researching this subject of free will over the last century. We now understand that we do not have the level of free will that many of us believe we do. Our decisions are determined by genetics, upbringing, society, media, political climate and lived experiences, including prejudices and biases. An individual's decisions are not of their own making.

Regarding weight, how we choose to nourish ourselves should be done with an understanding of what's best for our bodies. Unfortunately, mass marketing and advertising seek to categorize the general public into a single group so that they can all be sold the same product regardless of race, gender, age, medical history, lifestyle or income. Organizations carry this out without considering the power they wield. This mass generalization is yet another contributor to the obesity problem. We need to wake up from the illusion of free will and replace it with the understanding that we are fallible human beings, susceptible to influence, mainly at the mercy of the combined impact of our culture and the society we live in. Once we view the world through that lens, we can begin to let go of judgement, the driving force behind all the stigma and discrimination. Accepting that we do not have complete control over our minds allows us to disassociate ourselves from the lies we have been led to believe. Instead, we are able to explore several possibilities that we might not have considered otherwise.

At a Glance

❖ The advertising and marketing of food products significantly influence food choices, especially among young people. Food preferences established from an early age and maintained into adulthood create a foundation for long-term health consequences.

❖ Advertising invades our minds—it aims to make people want a particular product, regardless of whether or not they need it. Contrary to popular belief, willpower is not an innate trait that you are born with. Instead, it is a complex mind–body response that can be weakened by many tactics employed by the food industry.

---

* * *

8

Diet Culture and Body
Positivity—Misleading Cues

The only thing anyone can diagnose by looking at a fat person is their own level of prejudice toward fat people.

—Anti-Diet Activist and Author,
Marilyn Wann

Do Diets Work?

Special diets have always been intertwined with our lives, either by choice or through tradition. For instance, if allergies are a concern, one would intentionally exclude certain allergens from their meals. Choosing to consume clean wholefoods while minimizing indulgences is, in essence, adhering to a diet. Throughout history, healers have advocated for specific diets to tackle diverse health challenges.

In Ayurveda, the term *pathyam* signifies the practice of avoiding specific foods based on an individual's health conditions, needs and circumstances. It involves tailoring one's diet to promote balance and well-being by excluding foods that might exacerbate or interfere with certain health conditions. In traditional Japanese cuisine, known as *washoku,* the emphasis is on food harmony, aligning ingredients and cooking methods with the natural flow of the seasons.

The term 'diet', derived from the word *diaita*, embodies the concept of a comprehensive and wholesome lifestyle that encompasses both mental and physical well-being.[1] It extends beyond a limited focus on weight loss.

The first recorded specialized diet in Western medical literature was formulated in the 1800s and was attributed to William Banting. Banting was not only a scientist and a physician but also a carpenter and an undertaker. Inhabiting a corpulent body, he struggled to lose the excess weight. His doctor encouraged him to exercise more, which he initially did, but it also inadvertently increased his appetite. In 1862, at the age of sixty-five, his sight and hearing began to fail. He was then introduced to an ear, nose and throat specialist, Dr William Harvey. Dr Harvey had been attending lectures in Paris explaining the role of food and nutrition in diabetes. He was particularly interested in Banting's weight, given that he was gradually losing his vision and hearing.[2] He instructed Banting to eat more meat and give up bread, butter, milk, sugar, beer and potatoes—foods containing starch. Within a year of his new diet, Banting lost almost 23 kg, regained his hearing and significantly improved his sight.

In 1863, Banting avidly wrote his diet's success story in his book, *Letter on Corpulence*.[3] His low-carb diet was the first of its kind and became popularly known as 'The Banting Diet'.

Banting's diet was revolutionary. He swapped a diet high in sugar and refined carbohydrate for one rich in lean protein and healthy fats, which we now know is health-promoting and was the reason behind his successful weight loss.

Since then, a tidal wave of diets commenced: Atkins, keto, vegan, raw vegan, low-fat, low-carb, ultra-low-fat, ultra-low-carb, no carb, detox, Paleo, the Dukan diet, the HCG diet, intermittent fasting, the Mediterranean diet, Weight Watchers, Slim Fast, Jenny Craig, the South Beach diet, the Zone diet, the cabbage soup diet, Volumetrics, Golo, blood type diet, even a *baby food* diet and the list goes on and on.

In 2023, during the eighteenth Food and Health Survey by the International Food Information Council (IFIC), it was revealed that 52 per cent of Americans adopted a restricted eating pattern (up from 38 per cent in 2019) i.e. more than half of the US population adopted a specialized diet.[4] Given that approximately 80 per cent of dieters fail to achieve and maintain long-term results, we know that 80 per cent of the 52 per cent of Americans were doomed to fail in their weight-loss efforts.[5]

Unfortunately, the underlying truth is that most of these restrictive diets are so limiting that the dieter's resolve gradually wavers. When they fall off the wagon, they might eat all they want and regain any previously lost weight. Some diets rule out entire food groups while others, like the detox diet, rule out solid foods altogether. Research shows that the best diet is one that includes a variety of nutrient-rich foods in appropriate portions, providing essential nutrients like complex carbohydrates, healthy proteins, fats, vitamins and minerals to support overall health and well-being. It emphasizes the right combination of foods from different food groups to meet the body's nutritional needs based on the season and location. The optimal diet is both healthy and one that an individual can adhere to consistently over time. Unfortunately, our society's mentality towards dieting has become warped and misconstrued. As a result, many people associate 'diet' with food restrictions rather than a lifestyle choice.

Diet Culture

The issue we face today is not exactly due to dieting. Instead, it is because of something much more sinister—a diet culture that prioritizes thinness over all other considerations, including health. It is best summarized by Kate Moss's now-iconic quote, 'nothing tastes as good as skinny feels'.[6] The government-funded war on obesity has only exacerbated the stigma that endlessly attacks those suffering from obesity, further compounding the stereotypes, fat shaming and harassment associated with obesity.[7]

Diet culture has promoted the perception that thin, lean and toned bodies are the norm, not the exception, and the food and medication industries have quickly capitalized on this trend. While in the past, it was widely said that 'sex sells', it has been replaced by 'thin sells' now. In our society today, individuals who can discount their bodily needs in pursuit of thinness are regarded almost reverently.

We've had the white privilege and male privilege, and we're now dealing with thin privilege. In an interview with *Good Morning America*, Cora Harrington, founder of The Lingerie Addict and author of the book *In Intimate Detail*, described thin privilege as 'a system of benefits or advantages that society gives you for looking or being thin'.[8] Of course, people living in larger bodies are excluded from these benefits or advantages.

Inequality is prevalent worldwide. Racism, sexism, ageism and sizeism are rife despite the tireless efforts of advocacy groups who speak out for marginalized people. While the pro-slimness culture is gaining popularity, we equally see the rise of a counter-cultural campaign: the body positivity movement.

> We've had the white privilege and male privilege and we're now dealing with thin privilege.

Body Positivity

In the 1960s, black women pioneered the fat acceptance movement, which was the first cultural pushback against fat shaming especially in public settings like the workplace and the doctor's office. In 1969, a non-profit organization called the National Association to Aid Fat Americans was established, serving to fight for the civil rights and acceptance of fat individuals.[9] It eventually changed its name to the current one used today—NAAFA, the

National Association to Advance Fat Acceptance. This organization was a driving force behind the fat positivity movement, which was started in response to the rise of fat shaming and fatphobia in the American culture.

In 1996, the phrase 'body positive' was coined with the launch of thebodypositive.org.[10] This website offered educational materials to help people feel satisfied about their bodies by taking off the focus from losing weight through extreme diets and exercise efforts. It was not until 2012 that the body positivity movement attained widespread recognition as we know it today.

Incidentally, this was also when social media platforms gained popularity as a mode of mass communication, surpassing the conventional media, TV, newspapers and journals. Modern social media outlets like Facebook, Twitter and Reddit bloomed between 2004 and 2006, followed by Instagram, Pinterest and Snapchat, which all emerged in 2010.

The body positivity movement started when a group of fat activists networked online through forums and chat rooms. They then extended their conversations to Instagram and Tumblr. The movement garnered the most traction on Instagram, where #bodypositivity had over 7.2 million posts—a number which is growing daily. Body positivity, popularly referred to as #bopo, became a global trending topic. Since then, everyone has jumped on the bandwagon—registered medical professionals, influencers, you name it—some with purer intentions than others.

The fundamental notion behind body positivity is admirable—no individual should face discrimination based on their size, shape, weight, gender or physical appearance. Every person deserves equitable treatment across all aspects of society. It's crucial to eliminate both financial burdens, such as paying for extra airplane seats, and the social stigma attached to being overweight or obese due to a prevailing pro-thin culture. Body positivity is about embracing and appreciating all body types.

Unfortunately, as with most movements, the body positivity movement also became a target for major corporations. As the idea gained widespread momentum, big corporations exploited it and used it as a marketing ploy. Worse still, it often became an excuse for poor lifestyle choices.

In 2004, Dove famously led the charge in profiting from the body acceptance movement with their campaign for 'Real Beauty'.[11] The commercial campaign advertised a skin-firming lotion with the slogan 'New Dove Firming: Tested on Actual Curves' alongside six 'real' plus-size women. Dove was advising women to be comfortable in their skin, but at the same time, was also encouraging them to make it firmer by purchasing and using their product. Even though many people noticed the irony, the project generated more than $1.5 billion in sales following its launch. Many large-scale companies decided to replicate Dove's marketing strategy.

This has led body-positive advocates and researchers to question whether a beauty brand or any brand, regardless of its progressiveness, is truly championing body positivity. Their concern lies in the potential to create a sense of inadequacy, prompting individuals to spend their money. Body positivity should not be manipulated for financial gain. Unfortunately, even individuals within the medical field sometimes leverage the body positivity movement to promote books or consultations in order to generate extra profit.

Another campaign emerged and quickly gained widespread recognition to counter both the diet culture and the body positivity movements—'Health at Every Size'.

Health at Every Size

'Health at every size' is one of the most popular movements in the US along with the body positivity movement. Unfortunately, the idea can be misleading, jeopardizing its well-intentioned goal. A severely underweight person is as unhealthy as a severely overweight person. Beyond looks and appearance, this is an internal, physical, biological and metabolic health issue. Severely underweight people are more likely to suffer from brittle bones, low blood pressure, amenorrhea, malnutrition and mental illness. Correspondingly, people afflicted by sick fat are more likely to suffer from high blood pressure, heart disease, type 2 diabetes and mental illness.

Body positivity may be well intentioned and while it is good to have these 'good vibes', we should never ignore the health risks associated with adiposity and imagine that we are 'not at risk' even if we are severely obese. It is understandable to cling to optimism as a form of encouragement when we face shaming from many corners of society, but that doesn't mean we deliberately give ourselves false hopes irrespective of the reality. In doing so, we neglect our emotions and adopt a coping technique that is actually unhelpful or even toxic.

The term 'toxic positivity' is gaining momentum in the media parallel to the body positivity movement.[12] Toxic positivity holds that you should always maintain a positive mindset, no matter how difficult the situation is. This belief is toxic for several reasons—it is unrealistic to expect someone to think positively regardless of circumstances; we are too complicated and multifaceted for that to happen. Besides experiencing positive feelings like happiness and joy, we also experience negative feelings like frustration, anger, sadness, grief and shame. By insisting on remaining positive at all times, we will be doing a disservice to ourselves. We need to acknowledge our negative emotions when warranted as much as we need to celebrate the positive feelings and experiences when they come.

> Our lives are riddled with inconsistencies. Society values thinness and health while encouraging us to consume more and overeat.

Toxic positivity is counterproductive and intensifies the pain on top of an already difficult situation. The person feels guilt and shame when unable to maintain a positive, upbeat mindset. It prevents their growth as well if they constantly pretend that the problem doesn't exist and persist on 'looking on the bright side' and having 'good vibes only'.

Similarly, toxic body positivity can be harmful too. People place a lot of pressure on themselves to love their bodies unconditionally, but is it possible to truly love yourself? Is anybody able to do so? When you see someone who may look perfect to you, you are likely to find faults in your appearance when you look in the mirror. Body positivity tells you to ignore any negative body image issues, which outright disregards your living experience.

Adding insult to injury, today's landscape of the body positivity movement is very different from the fat activism movement it started out to be. As the hashtags #bodypositivity, #selflove, #selfacceptance and their variants gained popularity, people with smaller bodies began sharing photos and selfies of themselves in their #OOTD (outfit of the day) at the gym mirror tagged the same way. So now, when you search #bodypositivity on Instagram, you are more likely to see thin, lean and fit people than larger-bodied people whom the movement was created by and for. Unfortunately, this made larger-bodied individuals feel marginalized yet again.

To address the toxic undertones of pure body positivity, many activists are now advocating for 'body neutrality' instead. This method focuses on health rather than appearances. They propose that you should seek to feel neutral about your physical appearance and love your body for what it empowers you to do. In principle, self-love without focusing on your physical appearance will naturally translate into behaviours that nurture your body. Rather than exercising to lose weight, we will exercise to improve our health. We won't 'diet' but we will eat well.

In a *New York Times* article, Kelly DeVos, writer and author of *Fat Girl on a Plane* states, 'I am a fat woman. Growing up, I was chubby even during my adolescence.' Kelly recalls being bitten by a spider and hospitalized days later due to a severe flesh-eating infection. 'It took me years of hard work to learn to accept myself, but I finally embraced the idea that my body was healthy at any size,' she says. At forty-one, she was diagnosed with type 2 diabetes, which was rapidly advancing. She was dumbfounded. 'How can I have type 2 diabetes?' she remembers questioning her doctor. 'Fruits and vegetables are staples in my diet. I walk and do Pilates. I thought you could be healthy at any size?'

The doctor replied, 'You're not healthy at any size. Unless you make some major changes, you probably have about ten years to live.'[13]

Kelly's prognosis for her health was devastating, but it enlightened her about herself and the body positivity movement. It made her doubt the movement's principles, which claim that one should not attempt to reduce weight because it always reflects the psychological toll of fat shaming. She realized that was fallacious because she could choose to love her body while losing weight to love it better.

In many circumstances, adopting this mindset will result in actual 'health at every size'. This simply means that you can be any shape or size provided that your body remains healthy and thriving, your internal processes are functioning properly and your organs can perform their intended tasks without difficulty. Someone who has trouble walking up the stairs, either because their weight is so low that they lack energy or so heavy that they can't catch their breath, is not healthy at any size.

We Need a Cross-Societal Seismic Shift in Mindset

We live in a world quite different to the one that our bodies are biologically and evolutionarily designed for. There is such an abundance of cheap, processed, calorie-dense food readily available to us at all times, coupled with our largely sedentary lifestyles, that if we aren't watching what we eat and consciously choosing to move and exercise, we are likely to end up gaining a few extra kilos.

That being said, unless we have been unable to find a store with clothing in our size, forced to purchase an extra seat on a plane or been turned away from in disgust because of our weight, we cannot begin to understand the depth of the damage being inflicted, mentally and emotionally upon people suffering with obesity every day. Most of us don't have to consider whether a physician's office will have a scale that can take our weight or if we should bring seatbelt extenders with us on to a flight. There are obstacles at every turn for people living in larger bodies, and a big part of the problem is that so many of us in our society believe that they deserve what they get for having allowed themselves to become overweight in the first place.

> There is no such thing as a one-size-fits-all solution. All of the diets you see on a market may or may not work for you. Nothing works for everyone.

At a Glance

❖ Diet culture has promoted the perception that thin, lean and toned bodies are the norm, not the exception, and the food and medication industries have quickly capitalized on this trend.

❖ Body positivity is about accepting and loving all bodies. Unfortunately, as the idea gained widespread momentum, big corporations exploited it and used it as a marketing ploy.

❖ Health at every size means that you can be any shape or size provided that your body remains healthy and thriving.

* * *

9

Ageing Makes You Gain Weight

You can't help getting older, but you don't have to get old.

—George Burns

'Let me offer you some solid advice,' quipped one of my patients in his seventies as he readied to leave the hospital post-pneumonia treatment. 'Don't get old', he jokingly said. His jest held a kernel of truth—ageing often arrives with diminishing vitality and an uptick in weight.

Experts recommend establishing routines like regular exercise, mindful calorie tracking and weightlifting (strength training), minimizing sedentary behaviour as we age.[1] However, the challenges that ageing brings, such as diminishing hormones, achy joints, hearing impairment, cataracts, dementia and more, can complicate these efforts.

Faced with the seemingly inevitable weight gain, one might wonder if it's even worth trying. Although age-related weight increase might appear as certain as ageing itself, understanding its underlying causes could help uncover strategies to mitigate its effects. In this section, I'll delve into the primary factors driving weight gain as we age and explore potential solutions to counter it.

1) Loss of Muscle Mass

According to Dr Donald D. Hensrud, associate professor of preventive medicine and nutrition at the Mayo Clinic College of Medicine, one of the significant reasons behind acquiring weight as we age is that we lose muscle mass at a rate of roughly 1 per cent every year.[2]

'It may be imperceptible year to year, but compare the amount of muscle mass in an average 80-year-old to that of an average 20-year-old and it becomes more apparent,' says Hensrud, who is also a medical director of the Mayo Clinic's Healthy Living Program.

The Basal Metabolic Rate (BMR) signifies the calories burned while at rest and is tied to our muscle mass. With ageing, our sedentary lifestyle tends to grow—less exercise, more driving, elevator use over stairs—which reduces our BMR and exacerbates the problem of weight gain. This leads to fewer calories burned and surplus stored as fat.

Hormones control various bodily functions, including appetite, metabolism, sleep cycle, reproductive cycle, sexual function, body temperature and mood. Hormonal changes such as a decline of testosterone in men, and oestrogen and progesterone in women can affect weight.[3] In women, oestrogen levels decline the fastest during menopause, which usually occurs between forty-five and fifty-five years of age. Oestrogen is essential because it lowers blood cholesterol levels, maintains bone health and protects the brain. In men, a drop in testosterone can increase body fat, decrease muscle mass, weaken the bones, change the cholesterol metabolism and increase fatigue, similar to what happens to women in case of oestrogen deficiency.[4]

However, it's a misconception to think that postmenopausal women gain more weight than males.

While both sexes gain weight, the decline in oestrogen levels in women causes a build-up of fatty tissue around the abdomen. This makes weight gain in women more conspicuous, reinforcing the perception that women are more prone to gaining weight. Furthermore, a decrease in oestrogen leads to a loss of bone mass, which causes discomfort owing to the decline in bone density.[5] Unsurprisingly, this dissuades people from exercising so that they do not strain their tired bones any further.

Weight gain affects both men and women in comparable ways. People tend to gain a pound or more during the holidays. This may not appear to be a significant amount, but when that weight is not shed for twenty, thirty or forty years, it accumulates.

According to Harvard Health, the synthesis of the human growth hormone (HGH) in the pituitary gland reduces in both genders around their middle age.[6] One of HGH's many functions is to build and maintain muscle mass. As HGH levels drop, it becomes more difficult for your body to build and retain muscle, which impacts how many calories you burn. 'It's a snowball effect,' says

Marcio Griebeler, MD, an endocrinologist at Cleveland Clinic in Ohio. 'You begin to gain weight, lose lean body mass and burn fewer calories, which adds up over time.'[7]

Strength training exercises can be used to help reduce excess body fat and increase lean muscle mass, which in turn helps to maintain healthy metabolism. You can do strength training exercises at home or in the gym. Here are some simple choices:

1. Using your own body as exercise equipment: Push-ups, pull-ups, lunges and squats.
2. Resistance tubing: Inexpensive tubes of various resistance levels are available in supermarkets or sports goods stores. They provide resistance when stretched and can serve as great tools for the home or gym.
3. Free weights: Start with low weights and build your way up. You can use any household item like soup cans, milk cartons, unused books and other slightly heavier items like weight equipments.
4. Weight machines and cable suspension equipment: These are usually available in gyms and might require some training before you start using them.

The solution to age-related muscle loss

To help with weight loss and sarcopenia (age-related muscle loss), experts recommend weight training at least two to three times per week, starting with 20–30 minutes per session.[8]

2) Lifestyle Changes as a Catalyst for Low Calorie Burning and Higher Stress

Apart from the decline in muscle mass and hormonal factors, lifestyle changes are also the culprit behind weight gain during middle age. Uncontrollable age-related weight gain starts long before we reach senescence. As people begin to have families, they often move to the suburbs and are more likely to drive to work instead of walking or cycling. In addition, the after-work hours that would previously be spent at the gym are now spent at home taking care of a toddler. Even if their child is older, parents no longer have any personal time to spend at the gym, practise yoga or go for a run. Instead, play dates, homework, sports training and general family life become the focus of their lives. Moreover, having already invested so much time and energy in preparing the food for their children, the parents themselves eat foods that are quick and easy to prepare, neglecting their nutrition intake.

Even if an individual opts not to have a family, they tend to have less time to focus on their health and well-being as time goes by, especially when their careers progress and their job responsibilities become more evident. This affects both men and women. As their careers become more and more demanding, people have less time to prepare healthy and balanced meals at home, and instead opt to grab whatever is available at the office cafeteria.

While a successful career offers numerous advantages, it also brings various drawbacks, including elevated cortisol levels (a stress hormone) in the body. Cortisol, is linked to fat accumulation through its role in promoting the storage of visceral fat, especially around the abdominal area. Elevated cortisol levels can lead to increased appetite, insulin resistance and metabolic changes that contribute to the accumulation of fat in the body. However, this doesn't necessarily mean that ambitious professionals have to give up their careers to prevent weight gain. There are several activities one can engage in to mitigate these negative effects.

The solution to weight gain due to age-related lifestyle changes

If possible, use a standing desk; take the stairs in the office rather than the elevator; incorporate a walk into your lunch break if feasible; focus on weight training during workouts since muscles have a high metabolic rate. Furthermore, do everything possible to prioritize sleep to allow the body time to maintain energy levels, repair and rebuild the muscles, ensuring that you are ready for your next training session.

After working more than 40–50 hours in a week, it is incredibly difficult to find the time or motivation to exercise. As a workaround to this, many experts are now advocating for HIIT classes (high-intensity interval training) a couple of times a week, a session of which may only last 30–40 minutes. It focuses on building muscle, burning calories and speeding up metabolism.

3) Prescribed Medications

As we get older, new health conditions such as diabetes, hypertension, depression, arthritis, sleeplessness, high cholesterol, heart disease, cancer, dementia and so on are more likely to appear in our medical records. The use of a few more pills often follow. What's alarming is that we may have to use multiple medications to treat a single ailment such as diabetes, high blood pressure or heart disease. In a cross-sectional study by the Centres for Disease Control and Prevention or CDC's National Ambulatory Medical Care Survey from 2009 to 2016 involving 2 billion patient visits, 37 per cent of people above sixty-five years of age were found to be taking more than five medications per day.[9]

A side effect of several commonly used medications is weight gain.[10] These include antidepressants such as Prozac, diabetes medications such as insulin, steroid hormones, seizure medications, high blood pressure medications, seasonal allergies medications such as antihistamines and so on.

Imagine, your doctor prescribes medications to manage an ailment and adds more as new medical diagnoses are added to your list. This list piles up and before you know it, you have already put on 10, 15 or 20 kg. You wonder why your weighing scale is cruel to you despite all the good things you are doing. You may not realize that the new medications may be the reason behind your weight gain.

> ### The solution to weight gain as a result of prescribed medication
>
> Consult your medical physician or pharmacist and ask them to 'deprescribe', i.e. find an alternative medication that does not cause weight gain.

4) Physiology

A 2019 study titled 'Adipose lipid turnover and long-term changes in body weight', suggests that the lipid turnover (removal of fat from fat cells) in adipose tissue decreases during the ageing process. As it slows down, it contributes to weight gain. Researchers studied the fat cells in fifty-four men and women for thirteen years, and all of them showed a decline in their lipid turnover rate.

Interestingly, based on the research findings by Peter Arner from the Karolinska Institute, it appears that fat tissue plays a role in regulating body-weight changes as we age, regardless of other influencing factors.[11]

Various age-related illnesses also make it far less likely for a person to maintain the same level of physical activity as they did when they were younger. For example, a condition such as arthritis results in pain that hinders an individual from keeping up with their previous levels of physical activity.

> **The solution to physiological changes due to ageing**
>
> While strength training (weightlifting) can help prevent age-related muscle loss (sarcopenia), its effectiveness wanes over time like any other form of exercise. Therefore, it's also crucial to maintain a balanced diet.

Not all aspects of ageing are disheartening. On a positive note, weight gain seems to stabilize after the mid-sixties for those people who tend to eat less as they grow older. According to the CDC, the obesity rate among those over sixty is around 41 per cent, compared to approximately 43 per cent for those aged forty to fifty-nine and 36 per cent for those aged twenty to thirty-nine.[12] Since an older person expends less energy, some conscientious people eat less as they age, which helps to prevent weight gain.

5) Social and Psychological Changes

In addition to physiological changes that come with ageing, psychological factors also contribute to age-related weight gain. The prevalent stereotype suggests that as we grow older, we become less energetic, weaker and less capable of engaging in the same activities as our younger selves. This perception often leads to reduced physical activity and more frequent indulgence in treats. This mindset plays a crucial role in how a person's weight may change as they age.

Additionally, it's important to acknowledge that those in their golden years have experienced challenges and hardships that are often unimaginable to us today. Many of them lived through times when walking or cycling to school and work was the norm, wearing hand-me-down clothes was common, and simple meals like bread and potatoes were staples.

It's also important to remember that this older generation lacks the same level of education as the generations succeeding them. Those in their eighties today were predominantly middle class and laboured throughout their lives. Only a tiny percentage of that group received a college degree. By the age of sixteen, most of them had dropped out of school. In 1965, only 12 per cent of men and just over 7 per cent of women had a college degree, even in developed countries like the USA.[13] Today, we need to work hard to educate the older members of our society on the dangers of adiposity and poor lifestyle, ageing hearts and joints in particular, as well as the types of nutrition that will keep them feeling healthy and vital for as long as possible, with the best possible quality of life.

Theoretically, exercise must increase with age to compensate for the expected gain in weight due to ageing. Unfortunately, the inverse association between ageing and physical activity cannot be denied.[14] Physical activity levels naturally fall, especially as we hit our sixties. As a result, our body's energy consumption rate slows down and gaining a few kg appears to be synonymous with ageing.

According to researchers, even in the most physically active populations, most people endure age-related weight gain as they approach middle age and beyond. With this in mind, it's easy to see how someone might believe that it's better to 'settle' and accept their changing body with all its limitations. However, we can do something to mitigate the effects of age-related weight gain and it doesn't mean running our first marathon or embarking on a new crazy diet.

Health experts advise patients to clock up to 10,000 steps per day.[15] The concept of 10,000 steps has a fascinating history. It began as a marketing tactic to sell Yamasa Tokei's first pedometer, dubbed 'manpo-Kei' (meaning 10,000-step meter).[16] Back then, research had not proved that taking 10,000 steps would improve one's health. Nevertheless, the gimmick worked. Millions of pedometers were sold worldwide to people with a goal of reaching 10,000 steps per day. Subsequently, research studies showed the health benefits of walking over 8000 steps. Whether you hit the magic number or not, moving more is the goal. This can be achieved by taking walks throughout the day, or doing house or yard chores. Similar to the metabolic compensation we saw earlier with fasting and jogging, your body compensates for the extra energy burned through walking by increasing your hunger signals so that you consume more to make up for the spent calories and keep the total energy in balance.

The relationship between exercise and weight loss is an interesting topic of research.[17] 'Exercise is a crappy tool for weight loss,' said Herman Pontzer, an evolutionary anthropologist at Duke University.[18] According to his study, traditional hunter–gatherers who walked several kilometres a day burned the same number of calories as their sedentary counterparts.[19] Changing your food is vital for maintaining a healthy weight, though adding steps to your routine also helps.

> **The solution to social and psychological changes**
>
> Ageing per se leads to a gradual increase in fat mass and a decrease in muscle mass. Physical activity helps improve muscle mass, while healthy nutrition such as wholefoods or plant-based diets help improve the health of fat cells, and prevent or mitigate metabolic diseases. To maintain mental sharpness, one should expand their social connections and continue contributing to the family and society.

* * *

The journey to old age is not easy and the pathway appears to be peppered with potholes. Weight gain seems inevitable and the truth is, it is. But the *amount* of weight you gain is something you have control over as well as the *kind* of weight you gain. The path, though difficult, is ours to choose. Just like we must choose to build a healthy, wholesome life for ourselves in our youth, disregarding society's unrealistic expectations and standards of beauty, we also must not let the excuse of old age be an allowance for poor choices.

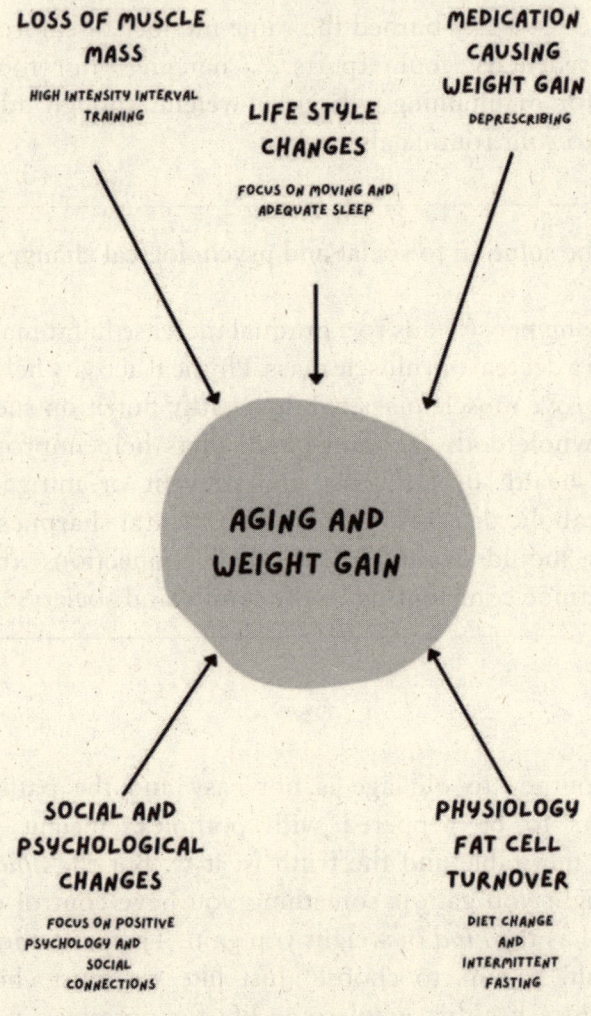

Figure 9.1: How to Maintain Healthy Weight gain with Ageing

At a Glance

❖ To help with weight loss and sarcopenia (age-related muscle loss), experts recommend weight training at least two to three times per week, starting with 20–30 minutes per session.

❖ Several commonly used medications have the side effect of increasing your weight. Consult your medical physician or pharmacist and ask them to 'deprescribe', or find an alternative medication that does not cause weight gain.

❖ While strength training (weightlifting) can help prevent age-related muscle loss (sarcopenia), its effectiveness wanes over time like any other form of exercise. Therefore, it's also crucial to maintain a balanced diet.

* * *

10

Role of Government Policies in the Rise of Obesity

Contradictory as it seems, malnutrition is a key contributor to obesity.

—Madeleine M. Kunin

The term 'Westernization' refers to the influence of American and European culture, science and businesses on other nations. In the 1960s, rapid industrialization in the United States led to a significant increase in food production alongside decreasing prices. By the early 1970s, obesity was emerging as a global concern. The suburban migration, the rise of refrigerator and car culture, and the growing availability of convenient fast food were all contributing factors. Simultaneously, reduced recreational exercise and more sedentary jobs were leading to decreased physical activity. For the first time in modern history, there was an excess of food supply compared to demand. While this shift was initially seen as progress in meeting human sustenance, it came at a considerable cost.

As the 1970s laid the groundwork for the rise of chronic diseases like obesity, diabetes and hypertension, epidemiologists scrambled to find ways to prevent diseases and promote the health of the population. More emphasis was placed on health promotion and disease prevention, rather than simply treating diseases and illnesses as they arose. For decades, medical professionals focused on three levels of prevention strategies: primary, secondary and tertiary. In 1978, however, a fourth level was introduced in response to the nation's growing health concerns— primordial prevention. Rather than focusing on the individual, as the primary, secondary and tertiary levels do, primordial prevention focused on altering the societal factors that impacted the weight, health and disease risk of a population.

Primordial prevention aims to reduce risk factors for the entire population through focused attention on societal and environmental conditions, i.e. ones that can be influenced through laws and national policy. An example of primordial prevention would be improving infrastructure that supports biking or walking instead of driving. Theoretically, as a result, risk factors for obesity, cardiovascular disease, type 2 diabetes, etc. would decrease. Despite the right intention behind this programme, its implementation was largely considered unsuccessful in addressing the burden of sick fat disease, as reflected by the rise in obesity rates.

The problem seems to be that even when policies are implemented, it's very difficult to change or influence people's behaviour. Sometimes success may be seen in small testing environments, but it simply isn't translating into nationwide change. In 2007, *Men's Fitness* announced Oklahoma as the eighth fattest city in America, to the dismay of Mayor Mick Cornett.[1] On New Year's Eve, Cornett summoned the local media and made an announcement—he was putting the city of Oklahoma on a diet. He admitted that it was a risky move, joking that he 'just put [his] wife on a diet' and that 'the city's residents needed to look more like ferrets and less like elephants'.

A website was created to track the city's progress as they endeavoured to lose a cumulative 1 million pounds (4,53,600 kg). Local businesses took note and the city's fast-food chains began to offer a 'Mayor's Special'. Cornett went on a morning news show with the head of the local Taco Bell franchise and even to his restaurant to hand out 'healthy' burritos. He knew he couldn't fight the fast-food industry and opted instead to work alongside the fast-food titans. People signed up on the website and began recording their progress, and in 2012, the people of Oklahoma City passed the 1-million-pound mark. After his bold New Year's Eve move, Oklahoma dropped off the *Men's Fitness* fattest cities list and Mayor Cornett was re-elected for two successive terms. Sadly, by 2023, Oklahoma has fallen to being the fourth most obese state in the US, with an obesity rate of 39.4 per cent.[2]

This goes to prove a couple of things. Governments *can* shift the social burden of obesity in the right direction.

However, if the might of policy is not greater than the temptation still being presented by cheap, tasty, calorie-dense foods, the success of the few will be mitigated by the continuing indulgence of the many.

In the 1970s, Bangladesh emerged from famine, with successive governments having worked alongside a vibrant non-governmental sector to deal with the underlying problems and visible symptoms of malnutrition among the country's population. Widespread targeted interventions were combined with a variety of nutritional measures to rebuild the health of the people, such as economic growth policies aimed at helping the poor, girls' education, improved sanitation and a significant turnaround in the agricultural sector, which moved Bangladesh from being a net importer of food to a significant exporter. As a result of these combined efforts, child stunting (the significant impairment of growth and development) fell from almost 57 per cent in 1997 to around 36 per cent in 2014.

Before the people of Bangladesh had a chance to celebrate their success, they were struck with an unexpected predicament. Rates of obesity among children and adolescents began to rise and have continued to do so, with childhood obesity emerging as a major public-health threat, in spite of undernutrition still being a significant problem. The people of Bangladesh are now shouldering the dual burden of both undernutrition and obesity, sometimes in the same household. A study showed that as people became more educated and began earning more, their weight increased significantly. This was seen profoundly among women, one of the demographics we know were targeted strongly with primordial prevention methods.[3]

In 2014, it was discovered that educated women were the most likely demographic to experience increased wealth, but also bear the burden of obesity. The student population of Bangladesh was also seeing a sharp rise in obesity rates. In a survey of third-level students, almost a quarter of respondents admitted to consuming fast food at least four times a week. Though 98 per cent of the students were well informed about the negative effects associated with excessive fast-food consumption, they were still profoundly addicted to it.[4] Kentucky Fried Chicken (KFC) was the first international fast-food chain to enter the Bangladeshi market back in 2006 and it primed the palates of the people of Bangladesh for what was to come. Today, Domino's Pizza, Nando's, American Burger, Pizza Hut and Burger King are all thriving, with Popeye's joining the ranks as of 2023, and those are only the international franchises.

It's easy to imagine the burden of obesity as being localized to the most industrialized countries, but we have already seen how even in developing countries such as Bangladesh, the fast-food industry, with its cheap, low-nutrition, high-sugar and high-calorie foods, is making its mark. In some countries, more than half the population is considered obese, not just overweight. The highest documented rate is seen in Nauru, where 61 per cent of its people are obese. The average weight of all Naurans is approximately 220 pounds (100 kg) and the average BMI is between thirty-four and forty-five.[5] Heart disease, high blood pressure and type 2 diabetes are growing concerns among the

Nauran people. In fact, on the island of Nauru, every other person has type 2 diabetes.

Much of Nauru's land is unfarmable due to approximately 90 per cent of it being covered in phosphate deposits, meaning the islanders are reliant on imported food products, the majority of which come in the form of tinned and processed produce. The diet of this Pacific Island nation's 10,000 inhabitants consists mostly of noodles, refined grains (predominantly rice), soda and processed food from cans. As Nauru invested more money in treating obesity, less money was invested in preventing it. Add to that the fact that culturally, Naurans view obesity as a sign of wealth, and as such, its people are happy to have sedentary lifestyles and have little to no desire to lose any of the weight that is also a symbol of their status in their communities, and it's not difficult to see why this problem has become so severe.

Nations strive to enhance food availability, ensuring an abundance of sustenance for their citizens. Today, with improved education and better job opportunities, an increasing number of people can afford unrestricted access to food. However, a pertinent question arises: despite the correlation between a country's economic progress and improved education, why are women, children and young individuals disproportionately affected by obesity, although they are aware of its associated health risks? Is it plausible that the population has consciously disregarded health advisories related to excessive consumption of unhealthy foods and insufficient physical activity, or is a more significant influence shaping this trend?

* * *

The designation of obesity as a disease marked a significant turning point in its history. This step was crucial in easing the burden for those affected, validating their condition as a medical issue rather than a personal shortcoming. This change aimed to dispel the misconception that obesity was solely a result of laziness or negligence.

Furthermore, the reclassification mandated insurance companies to extend support to policyholders in need of treatment for weight-related health issues, ensuring that healthcare providers would be reimbursed for obesity-related interventions. While this change brought about positive outcomes for those seeking care, it also carried unintended consequences that leaned towards consumerism and corporate interests.

The locus of control shifted from personal accountability to the medical profession and the healthcare industry, leading to a mindset that could encourage overconsumption and unhealthy habits. This outlook suggested that one could indulge in unhealthy eating with the assurance that medical interventions would address any resulting health concerns. From exercise programmes and equipments to medications and procedures, the avenues to manage weight gain expanded. The perception that insurance would cover all medical expenses further reinforced this approach.

As a result, we have become permanent customers to the collective market forces comprising ultra-processed food industry, health insurance and fitness industry, as well as the drug and device manufacturing industries. One industry feeds off another. Cheap food is purposely made to be as addictive and moreish as possible, in a manner that is desperately unregulated by governmental legislation, on neither the local nor national level. Instead of eating in an enjoyable yet controlled manner, many of us now eat mechanically without thinking, out of pure habit, because our society has normalized such consumption.

The distressing fact is that we all live in an adiposogenic environment created by the collective contribution of industry and policymakers. Sometimes well-intentioned practices and sometimes not, the common person gets swept in the winds of these collective forces and suffers. Many would argue that the consumption of the individual is no business of governments. They say that they can help to provide education and accurate information about how to make better choices, but cannot and should not try to *persuade* people in any way to do so. On the other hand, we know that governmental efforts can be useful—it was, after all, the US Surgeon General's report on smoking and its link to cancer that kick-started the declining popularity of cigarettes. When Dr Luther Terry made his announcement in 1964, almost 50 per cent of Americans, himself included, were smokers. By 2021, about 11.5 per cent of the population smoke.

As a society, we have total autonomy over what we put in our mouths and how we choose to nourish our bodies, but it would be remiss and reductionistic to assume that that alone means that we are immune to temptation. We all know that excess sugar and fat causes weight gain, and that processed foods are less nutrient-dense than a fresh equivalent. We also know that all of that 'bad' food tastes fantastic, is cheap and satisfies us in a way that steamed broccoli tends not to. When governments do intervene, change can occur. If ease of access is curtailed, people will be forced to make different decisions. In Arkansas (USA), an act was passed in 2003 which mandated that fast-food vending machines be removed from all elementary schools and students be weighed once a year, resulting in childhood obesity rates stalling. At the same time, if we compare the consumer price index of today with that of thirty years ago, fruits, vegetables and healthy foods are more expensive, while government policy has ensured that the prices of the raw foodstuffs that go into starchy, sugary foods have been kept low. It seems as though the governments are striving to make active contributions on a very visible level, but are failing to enforce meaningful policy on the back end, where big industries and lobbyists still occupy the driver's seat.

Governmental policies can guide and encourage, and do so successfully. They cannot be the be-all and end-all—a burger and fries is still a well-deserved treat that everyone should be able to access and enjoy. However, it is the governments who have the power to make fresh, local produce affordable on a large scale. It is the governments who have the power to mandate the provision of nutrition, education and healthy, balanced meals to be served in school canteens. It is the governments who have the power to remove advertisements for unhealthy food and drinks from daytime television. They have the power to improve health literacy and their country's food habits, the capacity to implement payment reforms, education and research. Only when these areas are addressed can an individual be blamed for the lifestyle choices they make that are contributing to obesity.

At a Glance

➤ A nation's food systems play a huge role in the health of its citizens.
➤ Governments have a large role in the health of the nation in general and the rise of obesity in particular.
➤ By changing policies, they can convert an obesogenic environment to that of a healthy one.

Acknowledgements

I owe a profound debt of gratitude to many, without whom this book would not have seen the light of day. First and foremost, I am immensely grateful to my editorial friends. Their relentless challenges pushed me to delve deeper, refine my ideas and persist in my quest. Their critique and encouragement were instrumental in bringing this book to fruition.

I reserve special appreciation for Harnoor Mann. During the nascent stages of the manuscript's development, her steadfast support and inspiration were my guiding lights. Harnoor's inputs were invaluable in shaping the narrative.

Clodagh Ní Fhaoláin deserves a heartfelt mention. Her unparalleled care and wise counsel throughout this journey have been both a source of strength and a fountain of wisdom. Her insights have enriched the content, and I am truly blessed to have had her on my side.

I cannot overstate the importance of Ngesa Oduor's role. Her meticulous attention to detail and dedication ensured that our labour of love came to a fruitful conclusion. She has been an anchor, ensuring that every word, sentence and idea aligns with the vision we set out with.

A special shout-out to Suhail Mathur, my dynamic book agent. With his expertise and dedication, Suhail has helped many authors realize their dreams of publishing their books. He turned the dream of publishing this book into a reality, steering it through the intricacies of the publishing world. His agency, The Book Bakers, has always tried to associate with the maximum number of publishers in India. I am lucky to have had him as my agent.

At the heart of any successful literary endeavour, especially at a prestigious house like Penguin, lies the silent and diligent work of exceptional professionals. My profound thanks go to Chirag Thakkar, my editor at Penguin Random House India. Chirag's sharp eye for detail, coupled with his constructive feedback, played a crucial role in elevating this work. Under his guidance, the book transformed and the best of it emerged more lucidly.

Aparna Abhijit, my copy editor at Penguin, stands as a shining light throughout my book journey. With an astute understanding of both language and content, Aparna meticulously ensured clarity and consistency throughout. I remain deeply indebted to Aparna for her invaluable contributions.

Last but by no means least, my deepest gratitude is reserved for my family. Their unwavering faith, endless patience and unconditional support provided the emotional bedrock upon which this entire endeavour rests.

Notes

Introduction: Obesity Is on the Rise—So Are Unrealistic Standards of Beauty

1. R. Puhl and K.D. Brownell, 'Bias, Discrimination, and Obesity', *Obesity Research* 9 (2001): 788.
2. S.G. Vari, 'Obesity: Rubensian Beauty Turned Into Major Health Problem', *Croatian Medical Journal*, 58, no. 2 (2017).
3. Alexandra Brewis, Cindi Sturtz Sreetharan and Amber Wutich, 'Obesity Stigma as a Globalizing Health Challenge', *Globalization and Health* 14, no. 1 (2018).
4. J.L. Lusk and Brenna Ellison, 'Who Is To Blame for the Rise in Obesity?', *Appetite* 68 (2013).

Chapter 1: Why Do We Stigmatize Obesity and What Are the Consequences?

1. 'Hispanic Children in U.S. at Greater Risk for Obesity than Other Ethnic/Racial Groups', *Elsevier: An Information Analytics Business*, 4 June 2009,

https://www.elsevier.com/about/press-releases/archive/research-and-journals/hispanic-children-in-us-at-greater-risk-for-obesity-than-other-ethnicracial-groups.

1. G.D. Foster et al., 'Primary Care Physicians' Attitudes about Obesity and Its Treatment', *Obesity Research* 11 (2003).

2. S.M. Fruh, 'Obesity Stigma and Bias', *Journal for Nurse Practitioners: JNP* 12, no. 7 (2016).

3. R.M. Puhl and C.A. Heuer, 'Obesity Stigma: Important Considerations for Public Health', *American Journal of Public Health* 100, no. 6 (2010).

4. M.Y. Poon and M. Tarrant, 'Obesity: Attitudes of Undergraduate Student Nurses and Registered Nurses', *Journal of Clinical Nursing* 18, no. 16 (2009).

5. R. M. Puhl, L.M. Lessard, M.S. Himmelstein and G.D. Foster, 'The Roles of Experienced and Internalized Weight Stigma in Healthcare Experiences: Perspectives of Adults Engaged in Weight Management Across Six Countries', *PLOS One* 16, no. 6 (2021).

6. Werner J. Cahnman, 'The Stigma of Obesity', *Sociological Quarterly* 9, no. 3 (1968).

7. A.J. Tomiyama et al., 'How and Why Weight Stigma Drives the Obesity "Epidemic" and Harms Health', *BMC Medicine* 16, no. 1 (2018).

8. A. Gandra, 'In Brazil, Body-shaming Most Common in Family Environment', Agência Brasil, 18 September 2022, https://agenciabrasil.ebc.com.br/en/https%3A//agenciabrasil.ebc.com.br/en/node/1481875.

9. G. Øen et al., 'Adolescents' Perspectives on Everyday Life with Obesity: A Qualitative Study', *International Journal of Qualitative Studies on Health and Well-being* 13 (2018).

10. 'Obesity Stigma at Work: Improving Inclusion and Productivity', EASO, 2 December 2022, https://easo.org/obesity-stigma-at-work-improving-inclusion-and-productivity/.

11. V. Tovar, 'My Weight Has Affected My Career', *Forbes*, 1 October 2018, https://www.forbes.com/sites/virgietovar/2018/09/30/my-weight-affected-my-career/?sh=277627cd139f.

12. 'Most Hiring Managers Will Not Even Consider Employing an Overweight Woman', City-data forum, last accessed 11 April 2023, https://www.city-data.com/forum/work-employment/2859771-most-hiring-managers-will-not-even.html.

13. W. DeJong, 'The Stigma of Obesity: The Consequences of Naive Assumptions Concerning the Causes of Physical Deviance', *Journal of Health and Social Behavior* 21, no. 1 (1980).

14. R.M. Puhl and K.D. Brownell, 'Bias, Discrimination, and Obesity', *Obesity Research* 9 (2001): 778.

15. R.M. Puhl and K.D. Brownell, 'Psychological Origins of Obesity Stigma: Toward Changing a Powerful and Pervasive Bias', *International Association for the Study of Obesity* 4 (2003): 213.

Chapter 2: Your (Average) Doctor Knows Very Little about Adiposity

1. 'Obesity and Overweight', World Health Organization, 9 June 2021, https://www.who.int/news-room/factsheets/detail/obesity-and-overweight.

2. 'Obesity', World Health Organization, 21 February 2020, https://www.who.int/health-topics/obesity#tab=tab_1.

3. G. Ndow, J.R. Amber and O. Tomori, 'Emerging Infectious Diseases: A Historical and Scientific Review', *Socio-cultural Dimensions of Emerging Infectious Diseases in Africa*, (2019).

4. J. Kagan, 'Annual Dividend (Insurance)', Investopedia, 11 September 2010, https://www.investopedia.com/terms/a/annual-dividend.asp.

5. Joseph Schumpeter, 'Origins and Evolution of Employment-based Health Benefits', *Employment and Health Benefits*, eds M.J. Field and H.T. Shapiro (Washington, DC: National Academies Press, 1993), https://www.ncbi.nlm.nih.gov/books/NBK235989/.

6. G. Jahoda, 'Quetelet and the Emergence of the Behavioral Sciences', *PubMed Central (PMC)*, 4 September 2014, https://www.ncbi.nlm.nih.gov/pmc/articles/PMC4559562/.

7. E. Faerstein and W. Winkelstein, 'Adolphe Quetelet', *Epidemiology* 23, no. 5 (2012); T. Rose, 'How the Idea of a "Normal" Person Got Invented', *Atlantic*, 18 February 2016, https://www.theatlantic.com/business/archive/2016/02/the-invention-of-the-normal-person/463365/.

8. M. Komaroff, 'For Researchers on Obesity: Historical Review of Extra Body Weight Definitions', *Journal of Obesity* (2016).

9. A.M. Czerniawski, 'From Average to Ideal: The Evolution of the Height and Weight Table in the United States', *Social Science History* 31 no. 2 (2007).

10. H. Blackburn and D. Jacobs, 'Commentary: Origins and Evolution of Body Mass Index (BMI): Continuing Saga', *International Journal of Epidemiology* 43, no. 3 (2014).

11. G. Eknoyan, 'Adolphe Quetelet (1796–1874) The Average Man and Indices of Obesity', *Nephrology Dialysis Transplantation* 23, no. 1 (2007).

12. 'Reports of the Scientific Committee for Food', *Commission of the European Communities*, https://food.ec.europa.eu/system/files/2016-10/labelling_nutrition-special_groups_food-weight_reduction-scf_reports_27_en.pdf.

13. '1980 Dietary Guidelines for Americans', *Dietary Guidelines for Americans*, https://www.dietaryguidelines.gov/about-dietary-guidelines/previous-editions/1980-dietary-guidelines-americans.

14. 'Physical Status: The Use and Interpretation of Anthropometry: Report of a WHO Expert Committee', *World Health Organization Technical Report Series* 854 (1995): 1.

15. H. Rosen, 'Is Obesity a Disease or a Behavior Abnormality? Did the AMA Get It Right?', *Missouri Medicine* 111, no. 2 (2014), https://www.ncbi.nlm.nih.gov/pmc/articles/PMC6179496/#:~:text=%E2%80%9CThe%20accumulation%20of%20fat%20in,a%20pathological%20or%20diseased%20condition.%E2%80%9D.

16. T.T. Samaras, L.H. Storms and H. Elrick, 'Longevity, Mortality and Body Weight', *Ageing Research Reviews* 1, no. 4 (2002).

17. W.T. Garvey et al., American Association of Clinical Endocrinologists and American College of Endocrinology Comprehensive Clinical Practice Guidelines for Medical Care of Patients with Obesity', *Endocrine Practice* 22, no. 7 (2016).

18. W.P. James, 'WHO Recognition of the Global Obesity Epidemic', *International Journal of Obesity* 32, no. 7 (2005).

19. T.K. Kyle, E.J. Dhurandhar and D.B. Allison, 'Regarding Obesity as a Disease: Evolving Policies and Their Implications', *Endocrinology and Metabolism Clinics of North America* 45, no. 3 (2016).

20. Ibid.

21. D. Verissimo, 'Modes of Body Absence and Presence based on Bodily Sensorimotor Telos', *SciELO —Brazil*, https://www.scielo.br/j/pusp/a/yjtzYMq5Kp JdQDy4LPrXcQM/?format=pdf&lang=en.

22. A. Le Tellier, 'Blame Nixon for the Obesity Epidemic', *Los Angeles Times*, 27 June 2012, https://www. latimes.com/opinion/la-xpm-2012-jun-27-la-ol-nixon-obesity-epidemic-corn-20120627-story.html.

23. 'Obesity Is a Common, Serious, and Costly Disease', *Centers for Disease Control and Prevention*, 19 May 2022, https://www.cdc.gov/obesity/data/adult.html.

24. C.E. Rosenberg, 'What Is an Epidemic? AIDS in Historical Perspective', *Daedalus* 118, no. 2 (1989), https://www.jstor.org/stable/20025233.

25. 'In U.S., Self-reported Weight Up Nearly 20 Pounds since 1990', Gallup, 23 November 2011, https:// news.gallup.com/poll/150947/self-reported-weight-nearly-pounds-1990.aspx.

26. E.A. Dennis, 'Founding, Early History and Transformation of the Journal for Lipid Research to an American Society of Biochemistry and Molecular Biology Journal', *Journal of Lipid Research* 50 (2009).

27. Emily Carlson, 'The Big, Fat World of Lipids', *National Institute of General Medical Sciences*, 9 August 2012, https://nigms.nih.gov/education/Inside-Life-Science/Pages/The-Big-Fat-World-of-Lipids.aspx.

28. D. Gallagher, 'Healthy Percentage Body Fat Ranges: An Approach for Developing Guidelines Based on Body Mass Index', *American Journal of Clinical Nutrition* 72, no. 3 (2000).

Chapter 3: Wired for Regaining Weight

1. R.R. Wing and S. Phelan, 'Long-term Weight Loss Maintenance', *American Journal of Clinical Nutrition* 82, no. 1 (2005).

2. K. Timper and J.C. Brüning, 'Hypothalamic Circuits Regulating Appetite and Energy Homeostasis: Pathways to Obesity', *Disease Models & Mechanisms* 10, no. 6 (2017); J.L. Wilson and P.J. Enriori, 'A Talk between Fat Tissue, Gut, Pancreas and Brain to Control Body Weight', *Molecular and Cellular Endocrinology* 418 (2017).

3. N. Geary, 'Control-theory Models of Body-weight Regulation and Body-weight-regulatory Appetite', *Appetite* 144 (2020).

4. M.J. Müller, A. Bosy-Westphal, and S.B. Heymsfield, 'Is There Evidence for a Set Point that

Regulates Human Body Weight?', *F1000 Medicine Reports* 2 (2010).

5. 'Endoscopic Suturing for Weight Gain after Bariatric Surgery', *UCLA Health*, 11 April 2023, https://www.uclahealth.org/medical-services/gastro/ies/patient-resources/endoscopic-treatment-obesity/endoscopic-suturing-weight-gain-after-bariatric-surgery.

6. B. Beck, 'Neuropeptide Y in Normal Eating and in Genetic and Dietary-induced Obesity', *Philosophical Transactions of the Royal Society B: Biological Sciences* 361, no. 1471 (2006).

7. J.M. Friedman, 'Leptin and the Regulation of Body Weight', *Keio Journal of Medicine* 60, no. 1 (2011).

8. J.M. Makaronidis and R.L. Batterham, 'Obesity, Body Weight Regulation and the Brain: Insights from fMRI', *British Journal of Radiology* 91, no. 189 (2018).

9. T. Kishi and J.K. Elmquist, 'Body Weight Is Regulated by the Brain: A Link between Feeding and Emotion', *Molecular Psychiatry* 10, no. 2 (2005).

10. A. Aoun, F. Darwish and N. Hamod, 'The Influence of the Gut Microbiome on Obesity in Adults and the Role of Probiotics, Prebiotics, and Symbiotics for Weight Loss', *Preventive Nutrition and Food Science* 25, no. 2 (2020).

11. C.D. Davis, 'The Gut Microbiome and its Role in Obesity', *Nutrition Today* 51, no. 4 (2016).

12. F. Magne et al., 'The Firmicutes/Bacteroidetes Ratio: A Relevant Marker of Gut Dysbiosis in Obese Patients?', *Nutrients* 12, no. 5 (2020).

13. P.J. Turnbaugh et al., 'An Obesity-associated Gut Microbiome with Increased Capacity for Energy Harvest', *Nature* 444, no. 7122 (2006).

14. T.P.J. Turnbaugh et al., 'Diet-induced Obesity Is Linked to Marked but Reversible Alterations in the Mouse Distal Gut Microbiome', *Cell Host & Microbe* 3, no. 4 (2008).

15. M.J. Müller et al., 'Recent Advances in Understanding Body Weight Homeostasis in Humans', *F1000Research* 7, (2018).

16. K.D. Hall and S. Kahan, 'Maintenance of Lost Weight and Long-term Management of Obesity', *Medical Clinics of North America* 102, no. 1 (2018).

17. L. Berger, 'The 10 Percent Solution: Losing a Little Brings Big Gains', *New York Times*, 22 June 2023, https://www.nytimes.com/2003/06/22/health/the-10-percent-solution-losing-a-little-brings-big-gains.html

18. D. Przulij et al., 'Time Restricted Eating as a Weight Loss Intervention in Adults with Obesity', *PLOS One* 16, no. 1 (2021).

19. N.M. Byrne et al., 'Intermittent Energy Restriction Improves Weight Loss Efficiency in Obese Men: The Matador Study', *International Journal of Obesity* 42, no. 2 (2017).

20. A. Artese, B.A. Stamford and R.J. Moffatt, 'Cigarette Smoking: An Accessory to the Development of Insulin Resistance', *American Journal of Lifestyle Medicine* 13 no. 6 (2017).

21. Liu et al., 'Calorie Restriction with or without Time-restricted Eating in Weight Loss, *New England Journal of Medicine* 387, no. 3 (2022); D.A. Lowe

et al., 'Effects of Time-restricted Eating on Weight Loss and Other Metabolic Parameters in Women and Men with Overweight and Obesity', *JAMA Internal Medicine* 180, no. 11 (2020).

22. W.E. Barrington and S.A. Beresford, 'Eating Occasions, Obesity and Related Behaviors in Working Adults: Does It Matter When you Snack?', *Nutrients* 11, no. 10 (2019).

23. R. de Cabo and M.P. Mattson, Effects of Intermittent Fasting on Health, Aging, and Disease', *New England Journal of Medicine* 381, no. 26 (2019).

24. G.L. Tripicchio et al., 'Associations between Snacking and Weight Status among Adolescents 12–19 years in the United States', *Nutrients* 11, no. 7 (2019).

25. 'Clean Fifteen', EWG, https://www.ewg.org/foodnews/clean-fifteen.php, last accessed 23 September 2023.

26. More information can be found at www.cornucopia.org.

27. 'BPA in Canned Food: Behind the Curtain', EWG, 3 June 2015, https://www.ewg.org/research/bpa-canned-food.

28. G. Liu et al., 'Perfluoroalkyl Substances and Changes in Body Weight and Resting Metabolic Rate in Response to Weight-loss Diets: A Prospective Study', *PLOS Medicine* 15 no. 2 (2018).

Chapter 4: Weight-Loss Surgery—Far from an 'Easy Fix'

1. J. Neuberger, 'Do We Need a New Word for Patients? Let's Do Away with "Patients"', *BMJ (Clinical research ed.)* 318, no. 7200 (1999).

2. E.G. Clark, 'Natural History of Syphilis and Levels of Prevention', *British Journal of Venereal Diseases* 30, no. 4 (1954).

3. H. Emerson, 'Textbook of Preventive Medicine', *American Journal of Public Health and the Nations Health* 43, no. 6 (1953).

4. Walter J. Pories et al., 'Is Type II Diabetes Mellitus (NIDDM) a Surgical Disease?', *Annals of Surgery* 215, no. 6 (1992).

5. W.J. Pories et al., 'Who Would Have Thought It? An Operation Proves to Be the Most Effective Therapy for Adult-onset Diabetes Mellitus', *Annals of Surgery* 222, no. 3 (1995).

6. 'About ASMBS', *American Society for Metabolic and Bariatric Surgery*, 11 April 2023, https://asmbs.org/about.

7. P. Neighmond, 'Weight-loss Surgery: It's Not for Everyone', *NPR*, 17 August 2006, www.npr.org/2006/08/17/5658690/weight-loss-surgery-its-not-for-everyone.

8. F. Biobaku et al., 'Bariatric Surgery: Remission of Inflammation, Cardiometabolic Benefits, and Common Adverse Effects', *Journal of the Endocrine Society* 4, no. 9 (2020).

9. J. Belluz, 'How Well Does Bariatric Surgery Work? We Asked 11 People Who Got It', Vox, 19 December 2017, https://www.vox.com/science-and-health/2017/12/19/16742884/weight-loss-bariatric-surgery-pros-cons-stories.

10. Ibid.

11. L.R. Vartanian and J. Fardouly, 'The Stigma of Obesity Surgery: Negative Evaluations based on Weight Loss History', *Obesity Surgery* 23, no. 10 (2013).

12. J. Belluz, 'How Well Does Bariatric Surgery Work? We Asked 11 People Who Got It', Vox, 19 December 2017, https://www.vox.com/science-and-health/2017/12/19/16742884/weight-loss-bariatric-surgery-pros-cons-stories.

13. P. Dolan et al., 'Assessment of Public Attitudes Toward Weight Loss Surgery in the United States', *JAMA Surgery* 154, no. 3 (2019).

14. J. Belluz, 'How Well Does Bariatric Surgery Work? We Asked 11 People Who Got It', Vox, 19 December 2017, https://www.vox.com/science-and-health/2017/12/19/16742884/weight-loss-bariatric-surgery-pros-cons-stories.

15. 'Obesity (Excessively Overweight): Health Effects and Next Steps', WebMD, 11 April 2023, https://www.webmd.com/obesity/what-obesity-is.

16. 'Gastric Bypass Diet: What to Eat after the Surgery', Mayo Clinic, 13 October 2020, https://www.mayoclinic.org/tests-procedures/gastric-bypass-surgery/in-depth/gastric-bypass-diet/art-20048472.

17. 'Projects', WW Philadelphia, 23 November 2022, https://www.wwphl.com/build-a-healthy-body-image/.

18. 'I Always End Up Crying in the Changing Room Whenever I Try to Buy Myself New Clothes', Reddit, 11 April 2023, https://www.reddit.com/r/offmychest/comments/80gop6/i_always_end_up_crying_in_the_changing_room/.

Chapter 5: Are We Food Addicts?

1. M. Macht and J. Mueller, 'Immediate Effects of Chocolate on Experimentally Induced Mood States', *Appetite* 49, no. 3 (2007).
2. 'The Phenomenology of Food Cravings', Docksci, 31 December 1969, https://docksci.com/the-phenomenology-of-food-cravings_5f4e8037097c478c408b456b.html.
3. T. Yoked, 'Why You Should Never Eat Potato Chips with Diet Coke, according to Brain Science', Haaretz, 1 April 2021, https://www.haaretz.com/israel-news/2021-04-01/ty-article-magazine/.highlight/why-you-should-never-eat-potato-chips-with-diet-coke-according-to-brain-science/0000017f-decb-db5a-a57f-deeb0a480000.
4. B. Willcox, D.C. Willcox and M. Suzuki, *The Okinawa Program: How the World's Longest-Lived People Achieve Everlasting Health and How You Can Too*, Three Rivers Press (2002), pp. 86–87.
5. B.C. Field, O.B. Chaudhri and S.R. Bloom, 'Obesity Treatment: Novel Peripheral Targets', *British Journal of Clinical Pharmacology* 68, no. 6 (2009).
6. C. Crier, 'What Does Gluttony Mean? A Biblical Definition of Gluttony', Christian Crier, 15 August 2015, https://www.patheos.com/blogs/christiancrier/2015/08/15/what-does-gluttony-mean-a-biblical-definition-of-gluttony/.
7. M. Singh, 'Mood, Food, and Obesity', *Frontiers in Psychology* 5 (2014).

8. M. Moss, 'The Extraordinary Science of Addictive Junk Food', *New York Times*, 20 February 2013, https://www.nytimes.com/2013/02/24/magazine/the-extraordinary-science-of-junk-food.html.

9. 'How the Food Industry Helps Engineer Our Cravings', NPR.org., 16 December 2015, https://www.npr.org/sections/thesalt/2015/12/16/459981099/how-the-food-industry-helps-engineer-our-cravings.

10. A. Le Tellier, 'Blame Nixon for the Obesity Epidemic', *Los Angeles Times*, 27 June 2012, https://www.latimes.com/opinion/la-xpm-2012-jun-27-la-ol-nixon-obesity-epidemic-corn-20120627-story.html.

11. A. MacDonald, 'How Addiction Hijacks the Brain. Desire Initiates the Process, but Learning Sustains it', *Harvard Mental Health Letter* 28, no. 1, www.health.harvard.edu/blog.

12. H. M. Espel Huynh, A.F. Muratore and M.R. Lowe, 'A Narrative Review of the Construct of Hedonic Hunger and Its Measurement by the Power of Food Scale', *Obesity Science & Practice* 4, no. 3 (2018).

13. S.H. Ahmed, K. Guillem and Y. Vandaele, 'Sugar Addiction', *Current Opinion in Clinical Nutrition and Metabolic Care* 16, no. 4 (2013).

14. G. Gronchi and F. Giovannelli, 'Dual Process Theory of Thought and Default Mode Network: A Possible Neural Foundation of Fast Thinking', *Frontiers in Psychology* 9 (2018).

15. M.J. Kreek, 'Cocaine, Dopamine and the Endogenous Opioid System', *Journal of Addictive Diseases* 15, no. 4 (1996).

16. K.C. Berridge and M. Kringelbach, 'Pleasure Systems in the Brain', *Neuron* 86, no. 3 (2015).

17. L. Rapaport, 'Brain Chemical Dopamine Bounces Back After Quitting Smoking', *Reuters*, 11 August 2016, https://www.reuters.com/article/us-health-dopamine-smoking-idUSKCN10L2LQ.

18. B.W. Balleine, M.R. Delgado, and O. Hikosaka, 'The Role of the Dorsal Striatum in Reward and Decision-making', *Journal of Neuroscience* 27, no. 31 (2007).

19. K.C. Berridge, 'Pleasures of the Brain', *Brain and Cognition* 52, no. 1 (2003).

20. L.H. Epstein et al., 'Food Reinforcement and Eating: A Multilevel Analysis', *Psychological Bulletin* 133, no. 5 (2007).

21. S.E. Polk et al., 'Wanting and Liking: Separable Components in Problematic Eating Behavior?', *Appetite* 115 (2017).

22. S.L. Parylak, G.F. Koob and E.P. Zorrilla, 'The Dark Side of Food Addiction', *Physiology & Behavior* 104, no. 1 (2011).

23. C.F. Moore et al., 'Neuroscience of Compulsive Eating Behavior', *Frontiers in Neuroscience* 11 (2017).

24. S.B. Heymsfield et al., 'Hyperphagia: Current Concepts and Future Directions Proceedings of the 2nd International Conference on Hyperphagia', *Obesity* 22, S1 (2014).

25. O. Gruzdeva et al., 'Leptin Resistance: Underlying Mechanisms and Diagnosis', *Diabetes, Metabolic Syndrome and Obesity: Targets and Therapy* 12 (2019).

26. C.T. Montague et al., 'Congenital Leptin Deficiency Is Associated With Severe Early-Onset Obesity in Humans', *Nature* 387 (1987).

27. 'A Food Addiction Has Defined My Entire Life. And It Is Slowly Killing Me', *Guardian*, 2 August 2018, https://www.theguardian.com/commentisfree/2017/jun/01/a-food-addiction-has-defined-my-entire-life-and-it-is-slowly-killing-me.

28. 'After Ten Years of Depression, My Life Had Hit Rock Bottom', AEA, 14 November 2018, https://www.addictiveeatersanonymous.org/post/i-was-spiralling-out-of-control-2.

29. 'Our Epidemic of Loneliness and Isolation', hhs.gov, https://www.hhs.gov/sites/default/files/surgeon-general-social-connection-advisory.pdf, last accessed 30 August 2023.

30. 'How Do I Know if I Am Addicted? Emily's Story', Food Addiction, https://foodaddiction.com/2018/10/how-do-i-know-if-i-am-addicted-emilys-story-10-off-november-27-dec-2-intensive/, last accessed 1 October 2023.

31. A.N. Gearhardt, M.A. White and M.N. Potenza, 'Binge Eating Disorder and Food Addiction', *Current Drug Abuse Reviews* 4, no. 3 (2011).

32. 'You Are Not Alone with Binge Eating', Beat Eating Disorders, https://www.beateatingdisorders.org.uk/your-stories/you-are-not-alone-binge-eating/.

33. C.M. Grilo, V. Ivezaj and M.A. White, 'Evaluation of the DSM-5 Severity Indicator for Binge Eating Disorder in a Community Sample', *Behaviour Research and Therapy* 66 (2015).

34. A. Muele, 'Focus: Addiction: Back by Popular Demand: A Narrative Review on the History of Food Addiction Research', *PubMed Central (PMC)*, 3 September 2015, https://www.ncbi.nlm.nih.gov/pmc/articles/PMC4553650/.

35. A. N. Gearhardt, W.R. Corbin and K.D. Bromwell, 'Development of the Yale Food Addiction Scale Version 2.0', *Psychology of Addictive Behaviors* 30, no. 1 (2016); A. Muele and A.N. Gearhardt, 'Five Years of the Yale Food Addiction Scale: Taking Stock and Moving Forward', *Current Addiction Records* 1 (2014).

36. TedMed, 'Why Do Our Brains Get Addicted?', YouTube video, 27 January 2015, https://www.youtube.com/watch?v=Mnd2-al4LCU.

Chapter 6: Flawed Nutrition Science Screwed Things Up for You

1. R. D. Feinman and E.J. Fine, '"A Calorie Is a Calorie" Violates the Second Law of Thermodynamics', *Nutrition Journal* 3, no. 1 (2004).

2. J.L. Hargrove, 'History of the Calorie in Nutrition', *Journal of Nutrition* 136, no. 12 (2006).

3. J.B. West, 'The Collaboration of Antoine and Marie-Anne Lavoisier and the First Measurements of Human Oxygen Consumption', *American Journal of Physiology-Lung Cellular and Molecular Physiology* 305, no. 11 (2013).

4. R.E. Olson, 'Evolution of Ideas about the Nutritional Value of Dietary Fat: Introduction', *Journal of Nutrition* 128, no. 2 (1998).

5. G.A. Bray, 'In the Footsteps of Wilbur Olin Atwater: The Atwater Lecture for 2019', *Advances in Nutrition* 11, no. 3 (2020).

6. W.O. Atwater, 'How Food Is Used in the Body – Experiments with Men in a Respiration Apparatus', *Century Illustrated Monthly Magazine* 32 (1897).

7. 'How Do Food Manufacturers Calculate the Calorie Count of Packaged Foods?', *Scientific American*, 31 July 2006, https://www.scientificamerican.com/ article/how-do-food-manufacturers/.

8. 'Stop Counting Calories', *Harvard Health*, 1 October 2020, https://www.health.harvard.edu/staying-healthy/ stop-counting-calories.

9. J.A. Novotny, S.K. Gebauer and D. J. Baer, 'Discrepancy between the Atwater Factor Predicted and Empirically Measured Energy Values of Almonds in Human Diets', *American Journal of Clinical Nutrition* 96, no. 2 (2012).

10. 'How Counting Calories Led to My Eating Disorder', Shape, 11 June 2019, https://www.shape.com/ healthy-eating/diet-tips/counting-calories-fitness-tracking-eating-disorder.

11. Philip B. Sparling, 'Legacy of Nutritionist Ancel Keys', *Mayo Clinic Proceedings* 95, no. 3 (2020).

12. R. Meach, 'From John Yudkin to Jamie Oliver: A Short but Sweet History on the War against Sugar', *Proteins, Pathologies and Politics* (2019).

13. 'Children's Cereals', Environmental Working Group, 15 May 2014, https://www.ewg.org/research/childrens-cereals.

14. R. Hoffenberg, 'Christiaan Barnard: His First Transplants and Their Impact on Concepts of Death', *BMJ (Clinical research ed.)* 323, no. 7327 (2001).

15. A. O'Connor, 'How the Sugar Industry Shifted Blame to Fat', *New York Times*, 12 September 2016, https://www.nytimes.com/2016/09/13/well/eat/how-the-sugar-industry-shifted-blame-to-fat.html.

16. R.B. McGandy, D.M. Hegsted and F.J. Stare, 'Dietary Fats, Carbohydrates and Atherosclerotic Vascular Disease', *New England Journal of Medicine* 277, no. 5 (1967); K. Doyle, 'Sugar Industry Downplayed Heart Risks of Sugar, Promoted Risks of Fat: Study', *Reuters*, 12 September 2016, https://www.reuters.com/article/us-health-heart-sugar-risks-idUSKCN11I1QH.

17. C.E. Kearns, L.A. Schmidt and S.A. Glantz, 'Sugar Industry and Coronary Heart Disease Research', *JAMA Internal Medicine* 176, no. 11 (2016).

18. A. O'Connor, 'Study Tied to Food Industry Tries to Discredit Sugar Guidelines', *New York Times*, 19 December 2016, https://www.nytimes.com/2016/12/19/well/eat/a-food-industry-study-tries-to-discredit-advice-about-sugar.html.

19. A. Le Tellier, 'Blame Nixon for the Obesity Epidemic', *Los Angeles Times*, 27 June 2012, https://www.latimes.com/opinion/la-xpm-2012-jun-27-la-ol-nixon-obesity-epidemic-corn-20120627-story.html.

20. Ibid.

21. D.I. Jalal et al., 'Increased Fructose Associates with Elevated Blood Pressure', *J Am Soc Nephrol* 21 (2010).

22. J.S. White, 'Misconceptions about High-Fructose Corn Syrup: Is It Uniquely Responsible for Obesity, Reactive Dicarbonyl Compounds, and Advanced Glycation Endproducts?', *Journal of Nutrition* 139, no. 6 (2009).

23. K.D. Hall et al., 'Ultra-Processed Diets Cause Excess Calorie Intake and Weight Gain: An Inpatient Randomized Controlled Trial of Ad Libitum Food Intake', *Cell Metabolism* 30, no. 1 (2019).

24. 'Food Pyramid (Nutrition)', Wikipedia, 13 August 2023, https://en.wikipedia.org/wiki/Food_pyramid_(nutrition)#/media/File:USDA_Food_Pyramid.gif.

25. J.K Glassman, 'Dihydrogen Monoxide: Unrecognized Killer', *Washington Post*, 21 October 1997, https://www.washingtonpost.com/archive/opinions/1997/10/21/dihydrogen-monoxide-unrecognized-killer/ee85631a-c426-42c4-bda7-ed63db993106/.

Chapter 7: Your Willpower Can Be Easily Hacked

1. 'Obesity', Centers for Disease Control and Prevention, 16 November 2021, https://www.cdc.gov/healthyschools/obesity/index.htm.

2. G.L. Paley et al., 'Overweight and Obesity in Pediatric Secondary Pseudotumor Cerebri Syndrome', *American Journal of Ophthalmology* 159, no. 2 (2015).

3. S. Laporte, 'Wonder Bread: The Rise and Fall of an Iconic American Food', American University, December 2007, pp. 1–49, https://dra.american.edu/

islandora/object/0708capstones%3A86/datastream/PDF/view.

4. 'Governments Failing to Protect Child Rights by Not Restricting Junk Food Marketing', World Cancer Research Fund UK, 20 January 2022, https://www.wcrf-uk.org/about-us/press-releases/governments-failing-to-protect-child-rights-by-not-restricting-junk-food-marketing/.

5. 'Unhealthy and Unregulated Food Advertising and Marketing to Children', American Heart Association, 9 April 2019, https://www.heart.org/-/media/files/about-us/policy-research/fact-sheets/healthy-schools-and-childhood-obesity/food-marketing-and-advertising-to-children-fact-sheet.pdf.

6. Yogi Berra, 'Advertising to Kids and the FTC: A Regulatory Retrospective That Advises the Present', Federal Trade Commission, https://www.ftc.gov/sites/default/files/documents/public_statements/advertising-kids-and-ftc-regulatory-retrospective-advises-present/040802adstokids.pdf.

7. Joe Cardador, 'The Power of Gen Z Influence: How the Pivotal Generation Is Affecting Market Spend', ed. Skyler Huff, Barkley and Marketing Millennial, January 2018, https://www.millennialmarketing.com/wpcontent/uploads/2018/01/Barkley_WP_GenZMarketSpend_Final.pdf.

8. *Congressional Record* 151, no. 133, 19 October 2005, https://www.govinfo.gov/content/pkg/CREC-2005-10-19/html/CREC-2005-10-19-pt1-PgH8925-6.htm.

9. B. Sadeghirad et al., 'Influence of Unhealthy Food and Beverage Marketing on Children's Dietary Intake and

Preference: A Systematic Review and Meta-Analysis of Randomized Trials', *Obesity Reviews* 17(10), 945–59.

10. T.B. Spears, 'All Things to All Men: The Commercial Traveler and the Rise of Modern Salesmanship', *American Quarterly* 45, no. 4 (1993).

11. C. McLaren, 'How Advertising Works', *Ad Nauseam: A Survivor's Guide to American Consumer Culture*, ed. J. Torchinsky (London: Faber & Faber, 2009).

12. E.L. Bernays, 'The Engineering of Consent', *Annals of the American Academy of Political and Social Science* 250, no. 1 (1947).

13. A. Theaker, ed., *The Public Relations Handbook (Media Practice) 6th Edition*, (Routledge, 2020).

14. 'The Ringer: The Scientists Who Shape What and How We Eat', *Center for Health Incentives and Behavioral Economics*, 16 October 2019, https://chibe.upenn.edu/news/the-scientists-who-shape-what-and-how-we-eat/.

15. S. Cave, 'There's No Such Thing as Free Will but We're Better Off Believing in It Anyway', *Atlantic*, June 2016, https://www.theatlantic.com/magazine/archive/2016/06/theres-no-such-thing-as-free-will/480750/.

Chapter 8: Diet Culture and Body Positivity—Misleading Cues

1. 'Diet', Etymology, https://www.etymonline.com/word/diet, last accessed 11 April 2023.

2. '150 Years of Dieting Fads: An American Story', CBS News, 25 January 2011, https://www.cbsnews.com/news/150-years-of-dieting-fads-an-american-story/.

3. W. Banting, 'Letter on Corpulence, Addressed to the Public', *Obesity Research* 1, no. 2 (1993).

4. '2020 Food and Health Survey', International Food Information Council, 23 May 2023, https://foodinsight.org/wp-content/uploads/2020/06/2020-Food-and-Health-Survey-.pdf, last accessed 11 April 2023.

5. Ibid.

6. 'Kate Moss Regrets "Nothing Tastes as Good as Skinny Feels" Comment', BBC News, 14 September 2018, https://www.bbc.com/news/newsbeat-45522714.

7. D. Mozaffarian et al., 'Role of Government Policy in Nutrition—Barriers to and Opportunities for Healthier Eating', *BMJ* (2018).

8. A. Vagianos, 'Yes, "Thin Privilege" Exists. This Viral Twitter Thread Explains It Perfectly', *HuffPost*, 11 April 2023, https://www.huffpost.com/entry/yes-thin-privelege-exists-and-this-viral-twitter-thread-explains-it-perfectly_n_5b5749d3e4b0fd5c73c9465d.

9. D. Fletcher, 'The Fat-acceptance Movement', *Time*, 31 July 2009, https://content.time.com/time/nation/article/0,8599,1913858,00.html.

10. 'About Us', The Body Positive, 18 January 2023, https://thebodypositive.org/about-us/.

11. Peitho Editorial Team, *CFSHRC*, 14 December 2020, https://cfshrc.org/article/the-dove-campaign-for-real-beauty-an-embodiment-of-postracial-rhetoric/; J. Millard 'Performing Beauty: Dove's "Real Beauty" Campaign', *Symbolic Interaction* 32, no. 2 (2009).

12. Elizabeth Bernstein, 'Toxic Positivity Is Very Real, and Very Annoying', *Wall Street Journal*,

2   November   2021,   https://www.wsj.com/articles/
tired-of-being-told-cheer-up-the-problem-of-toxic-
positivity-11635858001.

13. Kelly De Vos, 'The Problem with Body Positivity',
New York Times, 29 May 2018, https://www.
nytimes.com/2018/05/29/opinion/weight-loss-body-
positivity.html.

Chapter 9: Ageing Makes You Gain Weight

1. J.M. Rippe, 'Lifestyle Medicine: The Health
Promoting Power of Daily Habits and Practices',
American Journal of Lifestyle Medicine 12, no. 6,
499–512, 20 July 2018.

2. M. Cimons, 'Growing Old Doesn't Mean You
Also Grow in Weight', *Washington Post*, 27
October   2019,   https://www.washingtonpost.com/
health/growing-old-doesnt-mean-you-also-grow-
in-weight/2019/10/25/ccb0673c-ec2f-11e9-9306-
47cb0324fd44_story.html.

3. A. W. Van den Beld et al., 'The Physiology of
Endocrine Systems with Ageing', *Lancet Diabetes &
Endocrinology* 6, no. 8 (2018).

4. B. Lunenfeld, 'Endocrinology of the Aging Male',
Minerva Ginecologica 58, no. 2 (2006).

5. M. Ji and Q. Yu, 'Primary Osteoporosis in
Postmenopausal Women', *Maturitas* 82, no. 3 (2015).

6. 'Does Human Growth Hormone Slow the Aging
Process?', *Harvard Health*, 1 September 2020, https://
www.health.harvard.edu/mens-health/does-human-
growth-hormone-slow-the-aging-process.

7. M. Lawler, '5 Reasons It's Harder to Lose Weight with Age and What to Do about It', Everyday Health, 6 April 2009, https://www.everydayhealth.com/weight/weight-gain-and-aging.aspx.

8. M. Cimons, 'Growing Old Doesn't Mean You Also Have to Grow the Pounds', *Tyler Morning Telegraph*, 1 November 2019.

9. Eric H. Young et al., 'Polypharmacy Prevalence in Older Adults Seen in United States Physician Offices From 2009 to 2016', *PLOS One* 16, 3 August 2021.

10. 'Medications That May Cause Weight Gain', Obesity Medicine Association, 21 June 2017, https://obesitymedicine.org/medications-that-cause-weight-gain/.

11. P. Arner et al., 'Adipose lipid turnover and long-term changes in body weight', *Nature Medicine*, 25, no. 9 (2019), 1385–89.

12. 'Obesity Is a Common, Serious, and Costly Disease', *Centers for Disease Control and Prevention*, 19 May 2022, https://www.cdc.gov/obesity/data/adult.html.

13. E. Duffin, 'Americans with a College Degree 1940–2018, by Gender', Statista, 20 April 2022, https://www.statista.com/statistics/184272/educational-attainment-of-college-diploma-or-higher-by-gender/.

14. D. Fujita et al., 'Supine Effect of Passive Cycling Movement Induces Vagal Withdrawal', *Journal of Physical Therapy Science* 27, no. 11 (2015).

15. C. Maldarelli, 'Why 10,000 Steps a Day Isn't the Secret to Better Health', Popular Science 150 years, 26 April 2021, https://www.popsci.com/story/health/10000-steps-evidence-study/.

16. C. Labos, '10,000 Steps: Myth or Fact?', Office for Science and Society, 29 November 2018, https://www.mcgill.ca/oss/article/health/10000-steps-myth-or-fact.

17. 'Living Like a Caveman Won't Make You Thin. But It Might Make You Healthy', Duke Today, 17 January 2021, https://today.duke.edu/2019/01/living-caveman-won%E2%80%99t-make-you-thin-it-might-make-you-healthy.

18. 'Colloquy Podcast: Why Exercising More May Not Help You Lose Weight', Harvard University - The Graduate School of Arts and Sciences, 4 March 2022, https://gsas.harvard.edu/news/stories/colloquy-podcast-why-exercising-more-may-not-help-you-lose-weight.

19. H. Pontzer, B.M. Wood and D.A. Raichlen, 'Hunter-gatherers as Models in Public Health', *Obesity Reviews* 19 (2018).

Chapter 10: Role of Government Policies in the Rise of Obesity

1. A. Allen at al., 'How America's Top Junk-Food City Went on a Diet (and Fattened Its Economy)', *Politico*, 17 December 2015, https://www.politico.com/magazine/story/2015/12/oklahoma-city-weight-loss-what-works-213445/.

2. 'Most Obese States 2023', Wisevoter, 3 May 2023, https://wisevoter.com/state-rankings/most-obese-states/#:~:text=West%20Virginia%20is%20the%20

most,an%20obesity%20rate%20of%2039.4%25,
last accessed 1 October 2023.

3. T.S. Tanwi, Sayan Chakrabarty and Syed
Hasanuzzaman, 'Double Burden of Malnutrition
among Ever-married Women in Bangladesh: A
Pooled Analysis', *BMC Women's Health* 19, no. 1
(2019), https://pubmed.ncbi.nlm.nih.gov/30704454/.

4. T.S. Nipun et al., 'Bangladeshi Student's Standpoint
on Junk Food Consumption and Social Behaviour',
IOSR Journal of Pharmacy and Biological Sciences
12, no. 1 (2017).

5. Tom Tran, 'Obesity Rate by Country', FoodyData,
6 October 2022, https://www.foodydata.com/post/
obesity-rate-by-country.

Scan QR code to access the
Penguin Random House India website